Strength from Movement: Mastering Chi

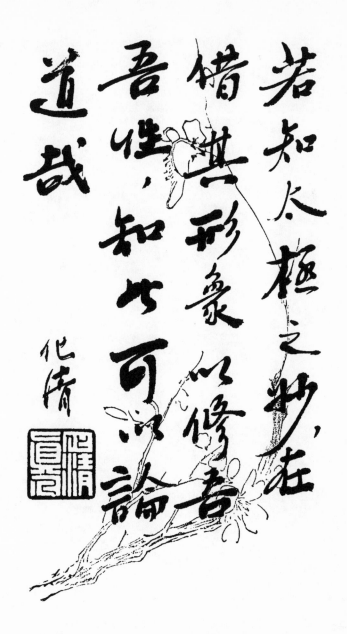

若知太極之妙，在
借其形象以修吾
吾性，知斯可以論
道哉

化清

The one who knows the depth
is able to use the form of t'ai chi exercise
to nurture the deep essence of one's life.

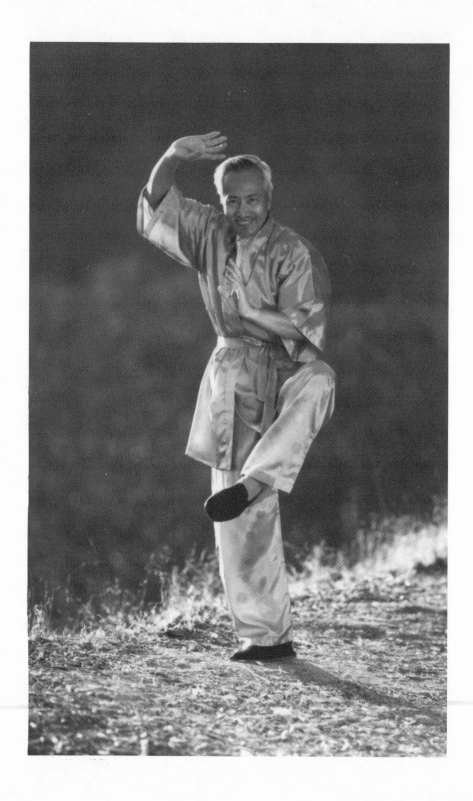

Strength from Movement: Mastering Chi

By Hua-Ching Ni
With Daoshing Ni and Maoshing Ni

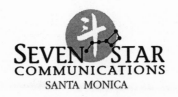

SEVEN STAR
COMMUNICATIONS
SANTA MONICA

The College of Tao offers teachings of many of the movements in this book, and about health, spirituality and the Integral Way based on the teachings of Hua-Ching Ni. To obtain information about Mentors teaching in your area or country, or if you are interested in teaching, please write the Universal Society of the Integral Way, PO Box 28993, Atlanta, GA 30358-0993 USA. To obtain information about the Integral Way of Life Correspondence Course, please write the College of Tao, PO Box 1222, El Prado, NM 87529 USA.

Acknowledgments: Thanks and appreciation to Rick Baudino, Suta Cahill, John Decker, Janet DeCourtney, John Rugis, and Tiane Sommer for their assistance with this book.

All calligraphy in this book was done by Hua-Ching Ni.

Published by:
Seven Star Communications Group Inc.
1314 Second Street
Santa Monica, CA 90401 USA

The paper used in this publication meets the minimum requirements of the American National Standard for Information Sciences Permanence of Paper for Printed Library Materials, ANSI 239.48-1984.

First Printing February 1994
Second Printing February 1996

Library of Congress Cataloging-in-Publication Data
Ni, Hua Ching.
    Strength from movement : mastering chi / by Hua-Ching Ni with Daoshing Ni and Maoshing Ni.
    p. cm.
    Includes bibliographical references (p.) and index.
    ISBN 0-937064-28-9
    1. T'ai chi ch'uan. I. Ni, Daoshing. II. Ni, Maoshing. III. Title
GV504.N5 1993
613.7'148--dc20
93-40503
CIP

Dedicated to those who enjoy gentle movement
as the art of life
rather than fancy martial arts
as a conquering force.

To all readers,

According to the teaching of the Universal Integral Way, male and female are equally important in the natural sphere. This fact is confirmed in the diagram of *T'ai Chi*. Thus, discrimination is not practiced in our tradition. All of my work is dedicated to both genders of the human race.

Wherever possible, constructions using masculine pronouns to represent both sexes are avoided. Where they occur, we ask your tolerance and spiritual understanding. We hope that you will take the essence of my teaching and overlook the limitations of language. Gender discrimination is inherent in English. Ancient Chinese pronouns do not differentiate gender. I wish that all of you will achieve yourselves well above the level of language and gender. Thank you.

Contents

Foreword

For those people interested in *t'ai chi chuan* for health and fitness, Taoism can be irrelevant. For those interested in its roots and highest goals, the principles are important.

It comes down to whether you are interested in chiefly how and what to do with your arms and legs and waist or whether you are also interested in how to live.

Achieving understanding is difficult because it has to do with how we try to perceive life and how we try to shape our lives.

In this issue Hua-Ching Ni discusses the Way and *t'ai chi chuan* and how to live.

Most of the important challenges in our lives are difficult precisely because we often do not really know what to do. And, of course, we have to do something. Frequently, these challenges are beyond our previous experience, or involve choices which are hard to make.

At one level, *t'ai chi chuan* helps us by providing enough balanced energy to approach problems with some degree of confidence. At another level, it can provide insight to deal with difficult choices.

Taoism, and similar sources of wisdom, share with *t'ai chi chuan* the capability to stimulate understanding and natural change.

Ni's message, in part, is to simplify life in order to make it rich and integrated.

The principles of *t'ai chi chuan* are very special in that they can help to integrate us into a natural balance with the way we have to live and the way we aspire to live.

Marvin Smalheizer, T'ai Chi Magazine
excerpted from "Editor's Notebook" of T'ai Chi Magazine

i

Preface

by Hua-Ching Ni

What's so great about doing gentle movement as physical art? It's so much fun to do!

The education of the Way is great. I have used it and benefitted from it. I was born with average intelligence and physical strength. Unlike a genius or a person of great wisdom, I needed to learn. In Chinese society, learning usually means studying books. However, broad reading is like hunting for a special object; sometimes you find what you want, but mostly you waste your time and energy.

In addition to reading, however, I was fortunate to have the physical and spiritual training left to me by my ancestors: gentle physical movement and the practice of spiritual self-development. Conventional Chinese scholars would find it hard to imagine that some simple movements could lead a wild boy with a restless mind and put him on the right path of a complete life, but those movements taught me the Way, developed my body, mind and spirit, and broadened my sense of responsibility beyond myself to include all of humanity and the universe.

You may wonder what the Way is. The word Tao or "Way," as I use it, has nothing to do with folk Taoism or temples. The Way that I adore and live by can be interpreted as a well-balanced, rhythmic life. Sometimes you are still and sometimes you are active. That kind of alternation illustrates the principle of *t'ai chi* or subtle universal law. We all live with the subtle universal law, and we frequently need to harmonize ourselves with it inside and out.

These forms of exercise, and indeed all kinds of movement, whether mental, emotional or physical are expressions of the subtle universal law. Thus, these exercises are one way to flow with universal movement through our small movements. They have become my impartial "religious" ritual. I do the simple movements of *Dao-In* early in the morning, and the movements of Infinite Expansion in the afternoon. This displays the unfolding of the universe. Thus, when I do the exercise, I am the universe. All truth is in my movements.

Confucius observed, "If I learn Tao in the morning, I will have happiness the entire day. Then if I die that evening, I will not feel regret for my life." I am sorry that Confucius did not have the chance to learn what I have learned and been able to pass along in my teaching, because he would have fulfilled his wish. If you try these movements, even one or two of them, you should have no regret over experiencing the universe as your own life.

All of my teachings have one core: the cosmic *t'ai chi* principle of the subtle universal law. The *t'ai chi* principle was the cosmological vision of the ancient achieved ones. No other theory compares to it. If you reexamine the first and second chapters of the *Tao Teh Ching*, you will see that modern physics comes close to it. Most people accept the creation myth from Genesis, but the ancient developed ones discovered the profound reality of how the universe began long before Genesis was written.

T'ai chi, or the subtle universal law, will be important in guiding advanced people in the future. My explanation of it in the book *Immortal Wisdom* [forthcoming] may assist you in finding your own proof.

Many people in this country age quickly because of the long hours they spend at the office or in front of their televisions. When mental activity is not balanced by physical activity, the coordination of the body is weakened. Too much food, drink, sex or work all have the same effect; thus many people can benefit from learning these gentle physical movements. I offer videotapes and books on four styles of *T'ai Chi* and *Dao-In*. They are suitable for people of all ages, and whoever practices them will achieve something beyond physical movement.

I hope you can use whichever of these movements suit you best to help your positive and virtuous life. Thank you.

Your spiritual friend,

Hua-Ching Ni
September 1, 1990
In the Mountains of Southern Oregon

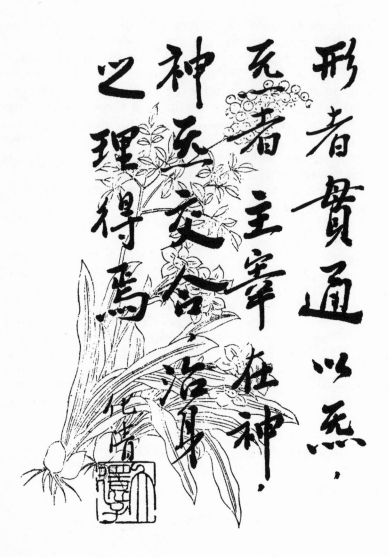

形者賢通以燕，
元者主宰在神，
神天交合，治身
之理得焉

It is chi which coordinates the body.
It is sen (spirit) which masters the chi.
When the chi and sen embrace each other,
    you are on the way to eternity.

Chapter 1

Introduction to Physical Arts

It is more important to achieve inner power than external force.
To win over people is to have strength but to win over oneself is to be
truly strong.   - Lao Tzu

Section 1: What Are Physical Arts?

I

Two Schools of Physical Arts: External and Internal

The physical arts[1] that are part of Chinese culture are of two schools: external and internal. The external school teaches regular martial arts that increase one's fighting skill and strength. Everything is on the external level of performance.

The internal school developed from external martial arts and may be used for self-defense in an emergency, but its main purpose is health and physical education and the refinement of individual physical energy. In other words, it can be described as a physical art for a spiritual purpose. What it teaches is not for display to others, but to strengthen oneself internally.

This is the basic difference between the external and internal schools. However, this classification is not absolute. Even people who learn to use or increase their external strength often find that they need a good, strong internal foundation, thus the external school also has internal practices. Yet the direction of the two schools is essentially different.

The external school, especially Shao Lin, is very popular in China, as is *karate* in Japan, *tae kwon do* in Korea, although the common source of all these practices is China. The internal school is appreciated by gentle people and a somewhat smaller number of extremely dedicated students who learn spiritual development from achieved teachers.

Typically, for any physical movement to survive and be promoted to young people in Chinese society, it must be a martial art. Young people want to learn something that can provide protection, so they are attracted to quick attack and forceful movements. Internal practice is totally different. No force can be seen when energy moves internally.

---

[1] In this book, the words "physical arts," "gentle movement," "*Chi Kung (Chi Gong)*" and "*T'ai Chi* movement" are used interchangeably to describe physical *chi* exercise. These words all describe a series of movements, both internal and external, that directly activate or help a smooth flow of *chi* or vital force through the body. They combine breathing techniques, simple movements, postural training and mental imagery. *T'ai Chi* and *Dao-In* are specific types of *Chi Kung (Chi Gong)* practice.

The internal school, which originated from martial arts, evolved beyond external moves when highly achieved martial arts practitioners realized that true protection comes from good health and good energy and from having the wisdom to apply that energy correctly in the world. Lasting protection does not come from quick, forceful movements.

In northern China, some practitioners of *Ba Gua* are very forceful and can defend themselves or attack others if they wish. This is the fundamental motive underlying their practice. The internal school, on the other hand, is like a walking stick that you automatically know how to use if you need to. Physical movement lays down the principle, but the learning is spiritual. This focus produces an entirely different result than martial arts, namely evenness, balance, smoothness, kindness, openness, harmlessness and generosity. These virtues can guide your life to high and beautiful fulfillment rather than toward the destructive skill of killing.

Detailed explanations of *Chi Kung (Chi Gong)*, *T'ai Chi*, *Dao-In*, *Ba Gua* and other arts, including an explanation of their similarities and their differences, is given in Chapters 2 and 3.

Section 2: Why Practice Physical Arts?

I

Gentle Physical Movement Enlivens You

When you dance, sing a song or listen to a funny joke, you feel enlivened or younger. Dancing, singing or painting naturally affect your emotions and indirectly aid your internal system.

However, the practice of gentle physical movement does even more to enliven and invigorate you than the arts. It works directly on your internal harmonization and adjustment. This is why, as you become more balanced, you also feel great pleasure. Gentle movement like *t'ai chi* and *chi kung* (also spelled *chi gong* or *qi gong*) has a self-generating, rejuvenating, lubricating (by stimulating all types of internal secretions) and refreshing effect.

If you consistently practice gentle movement, you will refresh yourself internally all the time. Whether you do it each morning or evening, or both morning and evening, and whether you do the whole set, half of the set, or even repeat just one movement, it is all beneficial.

A baby's entire body is light, soft and supple. Each muscle, tendon and bone has the resilience of the tender new life within.

Gentle movement refreshes you so that your body feels like a baby's.

People who do this exercise may seem to age just like everybody else, but they are internally different. They are refreshed clear down to the marrow of their bones, which actually slows down the aging process.

II

Physical Training

Bruce Lee, a young practitioner of Chinese martial arts, introduced these arts to the West and made them popular. Seeing this, the Chinese renewed their own interest in the old physical arts.

Self-defense is instinctual in all animals and it is a side effect of the internal school. The benefit of these arts is like that of a walking stick when climbing a steep mountain. You can make your way by using your hands only, but the walking stick makes the climb easier, and if the end of the stick has a hook on it, then you can use it to support you at the right time.

In ancient times, external schools had a simple requirement for achievement: if you had strong muscles, you were a good fighter and a winner of competitions. Physical strength can certainly do many things, but if you want to learn how to expand your energy and apply it, or if you want to experience a different sphere of life that is intangible and everlasting, internal *chi* movement is perhaps the best way to achieve these goals.

The internal school redirected the purpose of martial arts toward the internal practice of energy circulation. Circulating energy internally makes a person strong, thus one side effect of internal practice is to actually be a better martial artist.

There is another difference between martial arts and gentle movement. Martial arts psychologically prepare you to fight, but in gentle *T'ai Chi* movement, there is no rival other than yourself. When you bring yourself together in one piece using these highly developed physical arts, you achieve balance, poise and self-confidence and become non-aggressive.

We consider traditional *T'ai Chi* or *Chi Kung* (*Chi Gong*) practices as physical arts instead of martial arts. Martial arts are less important in modern times, while internal physical arts are always beneficial.

III
Health Enhancement

Master Ni: In ancient times, around 4,000 or 5,000 years ago and even earlier, there was no formal practice of medicine. One early remedy for physical problems was *Dao-In* (also spelled *Do-In*), which can be translated as "physical energy conducting." *Dao-In* movements can help minor problems in a short time. For example, if you have a sore muscle, you might try movement or massage as a way of treating it externally. This intuitive approach was different from the ancient healing ceremonies performed by shamans.

Gentle physical exercise can help you live your life in a healthy way. It is especially helpful for those whose lives are so structured that there is little spontaneity or flexibility in their schedules or their movements. Physical exercise is not something you do for others, it is something you do for yourself. More information on the health benefits of these practices is found throughout this book.

Dr. Daoshing Ni: In the early 1960's, many hospitals and medical colleges throughout mainland China began to study the therapeutic effect of practices such as *Chi Kung (Chi Gong)*. They used modern scientific methods and medical instruments to measure the physiological changes in the human body after *Chi Kung (Chi Gong)* exercises.

The Physiological Research Group of Shanghai First Medical College published a comprehensive report on the physical effects of *Chi Kung (Chi Gong)*. Some of the findings are as follows: a decrease in blood pressure (especially among those having hypertension), an increase of the skin temperature at the fingertips (indicating relaxation of the sympathetic stress reaction), increased mental clarity and overall relaxation, a decrease of the metabolic rate by as much as 19.7% - 34.0% during practice (signifying increased efficiency of metabolism), an increase in peristalsis (thus, promoting digestive functions), and an increase in appetite.

The most important discovery was that the nervous condition of the sympathetic stress reaction relaxed greatly and sympathetic impulses decreased. This indicates relaxation. This contributed to a decrease of the following: arterial pressure, cellular metabolic rates, blood sugar concentrations, and mental activity, and also relaxed muscular tones. After longer periods of practice, mental relaxation, ability to cope with stress, improved sleep, and a general energy increase were noted.

After the benefits of *Chi Kung* (*Chi Gong*) exercise were rediscovered, it became extremely popular among common workers and laborers, and *Chi Kung* (*Chi Gong*) therapeutic institutions started to spread throughout China. People with chronic illnesses eagerly rushed to the nearest *Chi Kung* (*Chi Gong*) institutions to learn this miraculous curing method.

There is a Chinese proverb that says, "When one has a chronic illness, one becomes the best doctor of that illness." This is true for Dr. Zhao, the composer of Crane Style *Chi Gong*. Since his youth, he was weak and sick, and was stricken with pulmonary tuberculosis in 1962. The drugs that he took did not seem to help, and his condition worsened daily. He was admitted to a rehabilitation center due to unsuccessful treatment at the hospital. One of his daily regimens at the center was an hour of *Chi Kung* (*Chi Gong*) practice. After eight months of continuous practice his condition had disappeared, and he was released.

Dr. Maoshing Ni: Some patients in Chinese hospitals practice self-healing eight hours a day.

Many studies have been done with *chi* exercise in China. They found that practice actually increases production of white blood cells within 40 minutes. If you take one blood test, then practice *Chi Kung* (*Chi Gong*) for 40 minutes and then take another blood test, there will be a jump in the number of white blood cells of around 25 to 30%. This indication of your immune system activity is dramatic and measurable.

With regular *chi* exercise, you will also find that you begin to catch fewer colds, but the benefits are not just physical. You also feel better on an emotional level because your energy is stronger. Your immune system is not just about exercising your physical body, but it is also about *chi* or energy which travels outside of your body and forms a protective field. Some people have a stronger field than others. A strong field helps protect you against the transference of undesirable or negative *chi*. This is important.

IV

Self-Control

Master Ni: Self-control is an important result of practicing gentle physical movement and one that enables you to avoid creating new predicaments for yourself. Instead of fighting and trying to control others, you are able to control yourself more skillfully. Even fighting is the art of skillfully controlling your own movement.

The true triumph in life is self-control, not the conquest of someone else. Soen Tzu, a Taoist strategist who wrote the classic *The Art of War*, said, "The high art of war is not waging battle, but making peace." Without fighting, you can still overcome trouble; better yet, you will be able to avoid problems in your life. Fighting usually causes even more trouble than you had in the first place.

Once you have learned self-control, and once you can skillfully control your own movements, you can arrange things in your environment so that you are undefeatable or invincible. You cannot be defeated because you can defend yourself well and your self-control is so good. By not defeating others, they win and you win also.

Physical movement is a spiritual practice that brings about self-development and virtue. Harmony is the virtue that results from self-control and appropriate action in all situations. This approach dissolves the sense of life as a battle and helps you rise above the pressures of the lower sphere of life. You learn to go beyond confrontation, contention, the network of worldly life and the engagement of emotion. You learn to go beyond a bad choice in a relationship, natural obligation, physical obligation and so forth. True development is not found in dramatic public performances but in everyday life.

V

Balance Your Personality and Emotion

Master Ni: Stagnant energy greatly affects people's health. When people do not know how to guide their energy correctly, they allow boredom to push them into wasting their energy through unnecessary or harmful pursuits. Basically, they do not know how to guide the energy of their mind and body at the same time in a good way.

If you take advantage of your free time by doing gentle physical arts, boredom will not kill you. Instead, you will make good use of the boredom. Exercise is also better than other kinds of fun that require money, travel or other resources.

Health is one of the benefits of learning and practicing gentle physical movement. The physical arts also help develop a well-balanced personality. When you attain balance between mind and body, you take a philosophically symmetrical approach toward all aspects of life.

VI
Stress Reduction

Dr. Daoshing Ni: Stress is an unavoidable part of modern life. *Chi* practice can counteract "burn-out" of the nervous system. The human body adapts to internal and external pressure by its "stress response" mechanism which causes the secretion of catecholamine, a neurotransmitter that tells the body to raise its blood pressure, speed up the circulation of blood to the muscles and increase respiration. The consequence of prolonged or sustained "stress response" results in being "stressed-out" or experiencing "burn-out" of the nervous system. Such stress can lead to problems such as high blood pressure, heart disease, muscle spasms and ulcers. The persistent practice of *chi* exercises counteracts stress on a physiological level and actually induces an opposite effect of the "stress response" thereby lowering blood pressure, relaxing muscle tension (especially around the heart), and protecting the stomach lining from ulcers by slowing down the sympathetic nervous system.

Chi exercise is an extremely valuable, if not necessary, tool to help our stress-filled society lighten the load on our already over-worked internal organs.

VII
Improvement of Mental Acuity

Dr. Daoshing Ni: Electrocephalogram (ECG) measurement of the brain waves of an ordinary person, taken when conscious, usually shows many inconsistent high-frequency, low negative waves. This indicates an unorganized and inefficient usage of brain capacity. On the other hand, the ECG of a person practicing *Chi Kung* (*Chi Gong*) on a regular basis usually shows consistent low-frequency, positive waves that are three times higher than those of an ordinary person. What this means is that *chi* practice can synchronize the electrical activity of the brain cells of the cerebral cortex and thus greatly enhance brain function.

VIII
Personal Enjoyment

Master Ni: For later practitioners of physical art, especially my generation, the definition of the internal school has changed. *Chi* movement is not only for gaining internal strength, but also for pure personal pleasure. My experience and purpose in practicing *T'ai Chi* movement is not to compete against someone else or to guard myself physically. I do it for pure pleasure. I am already confident that I can cope with situations, and I am already healthy. The four types of standing movement that I practice are the simple pleasure of my life. Sometimes I do it gently, and sometimes I do it vigorously, but never like the external school.

Some people take pleasure in watching movies, eating tasty food, reading an interesting book, meeting a good friend or doing other nice things. Practitioners of *chi* exercises can do those things too, but they have one more pleasure in addition to that: *chi* movement. Most people do not know about it, and that is why I teach it. The external school does it for show or fighting, but never just for fun.

When you learn the Way, you come to know that the Way is in everyone and everything. Applying the Way in your life makes your life fuller, more interesting and more enjoyable. The Way leads to good, productive fun, not the destructive kind of excitement that comes from drugs or alcohol. The pure pleasure and joy that come from your practice are more practical and lasting than other types of fun.

The secret to following the Way or learning *chi* movement is to enjoy yourself. The principle of Lao Tzu is *"wu wei"* which, practically speaking, means that if you are not too serious about spiritual achievement, you will achieve yourself naturally, just by continuing to practice.

IX

Artistic Expression

Master Ni: Let us take another point of view to understand this exercise more deeply. All gentle physical movements are a kind of art. All arts have a positive effect on emotional adjustment, but the best art helps you adjust yourself emotionally, physically and psychologically, all at the same time. When the subtle universal law expresses itself through movement, all of these benefits result, and your health is enhanced.

Artistic achievement is usually individual. It is not like printing identical copies of a book from a printing plate. Any art reveals your personal energy, but gentle movement reveals personal energy at a much deeper level than the fine arts such as painting, music, sculpture and so forth.

Good art, especially a spiritual or physical art, is esoteric. Some people talk about traditions in which secret teachings are passed down between teacher and student. In ancient times, because movement arts were practiced for personal rather than public purposes, few people could learn from masters. However, these exercises are now available to all. Even if you learn them for your personal enjoyment, they may also deeply affect your life.

Everyone needs to find something to enjoy. For example, many business people collect art. However, buying or looking at art is different from actually creating art. It is important for all people, young and old, to have a chance to learn some art.

Certain kinds of art are specifically designed to please people's emotions, and they have a certain value. Other kinds of art, like gentle movement, are not for show. You do not do it to please anyone or to get a response such as "Oh, how nice!" One of the values of gentle movement is to bring you back together in one piece so that your body, mind, emotion, intelligence and spirit function as an integral whole. If you do one thing and you think about another, then your movements will not be integrated.

T'ai Chi exercise is an art. It takes many years to make each movement meaningful, beautiful and graceful.

X

Longevity

Master Ni: The exercises I recommend in this book can be of interest for young people who would like to develop their potential in life. For people of middle age and older, the exercises are a way to improve their health.

When we focus on the subjects of physical health and longevity, it is important to remember that all life needs movement. The entire universe is constantly moving in all types of circles, big and small, horizontal and vertical. Any linear movement always comes to an end, but transforming a straight line into a circle makes it never-ending. *T'ai Chi* movement is a non-stop movement; you become inexhaustible when you do it. You never run out of energy or become worn out.

The ancient developed ones discovered that cyclic movement is the basis of the universe, with all the heavenly bodies always moving in their own orbits. That kind of discovery was inspiring to ancient people. It is one example of the way in which they learned from nature. One of the first things they learned from nature was to not cease moving.

In some cultures, people think that it is noble to be idle and have someone else, such as a servant, do everything for them, but that goes against the nature of life. We should value all opportunities to move, because natural movement promotes health and longevity.

During the Ching Dynasty, *T'ai Chi* became famous among the practitioners of all types of martial arts, because its approach was not that of brute force. However, those who turn *T'ai Chi* into a fighting tool pay the high price of shortening their lives. That is not the fault of the exercise itself, but the tension that martial arts champions create around it. It is not normal or natural to live with that kind of tension, day and night thinking about a possible surprise attack. Although such a practitioner may learn to relax physically, mentally they are still tense. The result is that they are soon killed, not by their opponent but by excessive tension.

Dr. Daoshing Ni: *Chi* practice can prolong one's biological potential. Studies have shown that after *chi* practice, changes in endocrine and neurotransmitter secretions become notable. Particularly, the prolactin in the blood stream increases along with a decrease in dopamine activity. Furthermore, the secretion of cortin decreases by about 50%. What this all translates into is a slowing down of the aging process and a strengthening of the immune system.

The health benefits of *chi* exercise are truly astounding. Surveys taken in China found that those who practiced any kind of *chi* exercise were much less prone to aging. Constant practice is the key.

XI

Inner Peace

Master Ni: When you do these movements, you enjoy both peace and movement at the same time. In such peace, you find all things in one. Peace can be alive, it does not mean the negative numbness of death.

Many people love sex, social glory and power, but none of those things can compare to identifying and uniting with the eternal

Tao or Way, which is what can happen when you practice moving your energy with gentle physical movement.

XII

Spiritual Growth

Master Ni: In addition to improving your health, the physical arts also guide you to refine your personal energy from coarse to fine to exquisite. When I was young, I had a special opportunity to learn gentle physical arts from my father's teachers and friends, who were very special people.

I have a great devotion to these movements, because they are a practical way to learn about one's spirit. If you pay close attention to what you are doing, you can learn something about spiritual truth by learning about its opposite, the physical realm.

Some monks take pride in being able to recite a few holy scriptures, thinking this can help their souls. However, a spiritually achieved person understands that continually repeating anything will deplete one's vitality and be of no benefit. A wise student will practice physical arts to attain a balanced view of life and a well-developed soul that is impartial and complete. The physical arts are actually a type of prayer for harmonization with universal nature.

Art is different from science. A scientific conclusion is not anyone's personal truth, but is a common standard. Art, on the other hand, is personal or individual. It can be common truth also, but it allows unlimited personal achievement. The learning of the Way is artistic, but it is also scientific. It is the process of discovering the common truth by dissolving the personal self, which is usually an accumulation of incomplete and distorted impressions from human life and culture.

To dissolve the self and restore our natural life, we learn practices from the healthy artistic sphere of life. When you become totally united with the movement, you dissolve your internal cultural distortions and are able to experience your original self. Each movement comes from the deep universal nature, which finds its expression through you. This art of life is, at the same time, the art of mind, the art of spirit, and the wordless expression of cosmic or universal law.

People usually enjoy sensory excitement or experiences of success. Gentle movement is a different enjoyment because it is spiritual enjoyment. Although it takes practice, once you achieve it you have a tremendous joy that cannot be compared to anything else. You find completeness inside and out. You find your "self" in each movement, yet it is no longer a narrow sense of self, because you join with the universe. Spiritual development does not happen by talking or by writing books; it occurs when you reach the same vibrational frequency as deep nature.

The most important element of life is the spirit. When you do gentle movement, you are not doing the exercise alone; all the spirits of your life are enjoying themselves. This is called "uniting with the great universe." During your exercise, there is no more separation, no more obstruction between the external and internal worlds. You feel the air around you, because your practice develops a special spiritual sensitivity. You feel the energy field outside and the energy field inside merge and integrate.

From movement, you discover the truth that the movement embodies cosmic law. You experience the universe revolving and evolving. You become a heavenly body, and you and the universe together become one united heavenly body. You unite with Heaven by always moving in cyclic patterns. All of nature moves with you, never getting stuck in any single spot. This is a high enjoyment in human spiritual life.

Scarecrows in the fields are stuffed with straw. However, wise people do not like to be stuffed with straw. They replace the "junk" that occupies too much of their time and consumes too much of their energy with ancient arts and skills that fill them with the high vitality of spiritual essence instead of consuming them.

XIII

Chi Exercise Enhances Healing Arts Practice
and Study Skills

Q: Dr. Ni, you are President of Yo San University of Traditional Chinese Medicine and you also have a successful practice of your own. Could you please tell us why an acupuncturist needs to practice T'ai Chi Exercise or chi exercise?

Dr. Daoshing Ni: *T'ai Chi* Movement and *Chi Kung* (*Chi Gong*) belong to a category of exercises that cultivate *chi* or energy. They also enhance one's vitality, prevent disease and produce longevity. For a practitioner of Traditional Chinese Medicine, these exercises can also enhance one's ability to provide better treatment for patients. It is very important for acupuncturists, as well as all health practitioners, to practice some form of *chi* development to enhance their vitality and thus their healing power.

Each movement of *T'ai Chi* has internal and external components, as well as *yin* and *yang* segments. Consistent practice of *chi* exercise teaches the health practitioner to become more attuned to their inner energy and more aware of their vital essence. With practice, as one refines and balances one's energy, it is common to feel exhilarated, balanced, and peaceful.

Most students and practitioners of Traditional Chinese Medicine in China learn some form of *chi* development. This is why it is required for students at Yo San University.

Q: Why is it important for a healer to have better, balanced energy?

Dr. Daoshing Ni: When a healer has good or high energy, the healing processes of inserting needles, hands-on touch and inquiry and diagnostic skills all tend to be more accurate. When a practitioner has good, balanced energy, his or her medical skills tend to be more refined and advanced.

If a practitioner has weak or scattered energy, their ability tends to be scattered and disorganized, and unfortunately is usually not as effective. Thus the practitioner who has higher energy is usually able to provide more effective treatment.

Q: From the standpoint of a student, will chi *exercise help my academic success?*

Dr. Ni: *Chi* exercises do not take that much time. Realistically, they require no more than an hour a day.

As we pursue academic achievement through intellectual development, it is even more important to balance ourselves by practicing *chi* development exercises. You will actually learn better if you have higher energy and more vitality.

Master Ni: Now that you know about *chi* exercise and movement, I hope you will learn and practice it. Everyone goes through different cycles at different times in their lives. The best friend you can have throughout all the cycles of your life is this practice. Sometimes ordinary people say, "I would be happy if I had more money." However, some things cannot be bought, such as the great joy of real practice.

Chi movement is the heritage of an unbroken spiritual tradition and must not be lost. Everyone can learn and use this excellent tool to achieve a long and happy life.

XIV
Master Ni's Experience:
The Movements Have Practical Value

Master Ni: I learned several styles of gentle movement from my father's teachers and those who learned with him. Most people know one style but never learn a second. I learned all the essential arts of the internal school, three *T'ai Chi* movements, Cosmic Tour and *Dao-In,* because my father's teachers and friends were kind to me. They knew that times were radically changing in China and if these arts were not taught, they would be lost.

First I learned *Dao-In*, Eight Treasures and Harmony/Trinity *T'ai Chi* Movement. As a boy, I was particularly attentive to those practices because I was not naturally endowed with great physical ability. Then, in order to develop stronger *chi*, I started to do the penguin-type walk of Cosmic Tour to strengthen my legs. I did it swiftly in the forest to see if I could keep my center of gravity low and still avoid hitting the trees. That training helped me become more agile, but I was unable to manage my movements in an ideal condition. Then I learned Gentle Path *T'ai Chi* Movement, which gently builds one's energy.

After practicing Gentle Path for some time, I felt that I needed to lighten and lift my energy from the lower part of my body, so I learned Sky Journey and Infinite Expansion, which are close to martial arts. In doing them, a person does not fight with anyone, but attains proficiency in movement. Essentially, you learn good control of your body's movements. Good movement brings poise and places a person in an undefeatable position in the first place.

I respect the art that I do. I continue to practice it, because it strengthens my physical being and leads to the attainment of an intangible, immortal life.

Many years ago some students in Taiwan asked why I made the decision to come to the United States. My answer was that only after the ancient arts are accepted by wise Westerners will the Chinese rediscover what they have devalued and neglected in their own culture. *Chi* exercise and spiritual learning have both started to generate interest in China now.

Section 3: *T'ai Chi* Movement is a Beneficial Practice

Master Ni's Talk at a *T'ai Chi* Camp
at Moran State Park on Orcas Island - June 3, 1989

Master Ni: Good morning. I am happy to meet all of you. Some of you are old friends, but most of you are new friends. This is a double joy.

I am happy that you practice *T'ai Chi* movement and are enthusiastic about learning it. It is also my own enjoyment, so we have something in common, and it is easy for us to communicate and understand each other.

T'ai Chi for Health

I recently read a report from mainland China in which two groups of people took a test. The first group of 15 older people were from age 58 to 65. The second group of 25 younger people were from age 18 to 25. Every morning, the older group went to a park to do *T'ai Chi* movement, while the younger group walked twenty minutes from their homes to a park to go running. The older people were at a general level in *T'ai Chi* movement, and some of them may have had illnesses or physical difficulties. They followed the instruction and walked to the park, which was good exercise, and then the instructor taught *T'ai Chi* movement for 15 minutes. They practiced a set of 24 movements, which were a simplified form of *T'ai Chi* movement. Meanwhile, the younger group ran one thousand six hundred meters (one mile).

One day, the researchers had both groups take some saliva from their mouths before and after their exercise to test the body's reaction to the different kinds of exercise. In the *T'ai Chi* group, the researchers discovered that two-thirds of the people showed an increase in a kind of immune protein called SIGA. That immune protein helps people be healthy, strong, and look young. Thus the older people, after walking and practicing 15 minutes of *T'ai Chi* movement, increased their immune power. For the young ones who ran, the saliva test showed that the immune protein, SIGA, decreased.

When you do *T'ai Chi* practice, you should keep the tip of your tongue touching the upper palate. This connects the internal channels of the body and enhances the internal circulation of energy. If the joggers had touched their tongues to their palates and given up drinking soft drinks, you might expect the results to be the same as those of the *T'ai Chi* practitioners. But the speed and mechanical repetition of jogging cannot produce the same results as gentle movement. Jogging is a fiery sport.

The internal practice of holding the tongue up is not only for exercise but is good to do in general circumstances as well. A bridge is formed by holding up the tongue. Talking or drinking too much breaks that energy connection.

The *T'ai Chi* Principle

Master Ni: The second thing we need to talk about is spirituality, which is different from religion. Even if no one here belongs to a religion, each of us has a spiritual life. It is not necessary to be a fanatic. If you are serious about religion, you may wonder, "If the Way is not a religion, what is the teaching of the Way? Why do people call you a Taoist Master?"

Tao is not a religion. The Integral Way is above all religions. It is the plain spiritual truth of nature. Unlike religions, which function at the emotional or conceptual level without ever reaching the subtle core of spiritual truth, the ancient spiritual teachings hold the key that can unlock all doors leading to truth.

The basic principle of the teaching of the Way is the principle of *t'ai chi*. *T'ai chi* as a principle is somewhat different from *T'ai Chi* movement. *T'ai Chi* movement demonstrates the cosmic principle of *t'ai chi*. When we practice *T'ai Chi* movement we benefit from the *t'ai chi* principle and can apply our learning in our daily contact with everyone and everything.

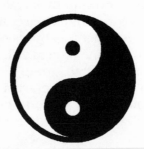

The *T'ai Chi* Symbol or Diagram

The principle or philosophy of *t'ai chi* started simply. Approximately ten thousand years ago, people's consciousness started to grow. Although it was not fully developed intellectually, there was an awareness of the difference between night and day, male and female, etc. As people continued to develop, they discovered that everything has two opposing sides, which they called *yin* and *yang*. On a mountain, one side faces south and the other faces north, and the vegetation is different on each side. In this way, a mountain also has a *yin* and a *yang*.

Humans have a top and a bottom. The top is *yang* and the bottom is *yin*. You also have a right side and a left side. The left side is *yang* and the right side is *yin*. Similarly, the front is *yin* and the back is *yang*.

T'ai chi is the principle of unity; *yin* and *yang* are its manifestations. Without *yin* and *yang*, the unity cannot be seen. If you are aware of this principle, you will notice that whenever a person starts to move or do something, their movement creates a discrimination between *yin* and *yang*. For example, when we are walking, our left and right legs alternate to keep us moving. That is the basic interpretation of *t'ai chi*. Both sides, help each other. If a thing stays still and does not reach the conscious level, there is unity or integralness, and you do not differentiate its parts.

In personal relationships of any kind, there is always an interplay of *yin* and *yang*. If harmony is produced, then it is a positive situation. If one side overextends itself, then imbalance, disharmony or destruction will be seen. To manage our lives well, we need to achieve *t'ai chi* or balance. Imbalance and disharmony go against the principle of *t'ai chi*, and anything that goes against the principle of *t'ai chi* will fail, decline and end, unless balance and harmony are restored.

The unity and harmony of *t'ai chi* are expressed when: 1) your mind does not fight your spirit, 2) your spirit does not fight your mind, 3) your body does not fight your mind, and 4) your physical desire does not fight your mind.

An individual person is a small model of *t'ai chi*, internally and externally. When there is disharmony, you lose your balance and disturb the natural balance of *t'ai chi*. It is important to be aware when that happens.

In *T'ai Chi* practice, always watch how your energy is flowing. Is it flowing well or not? If one part of the body or one movement is overextended, it creates a blockage in your energy flow. Blockage indicates imbalance, and you must correct yourself to follow the principle of *t'ai chi*.

Conceptual and ideological conflicts are common in today's world, but they are superficial and reflect nothing other than narrowmindedness. The human basics are: "I am a *t'ai chi*, and the world is a *t'ai chi*. Are things in order between me and society?" If there is harmony and balance, *t'ai chi* is there; you will be happy with your environment, and your environment will be happy too. When anything differs from this, there is difficulty and something needs to be corrected.

The most important thing in your *T'ai Chi* practice is to observe that when your outside moves, is the inside moving too? If the inside is not moving, then you are not unified. Even without unifying themselves inside, ambitious leaders say, "I am going to unify the whole world!" That is a fantasy. It cannot be that way.

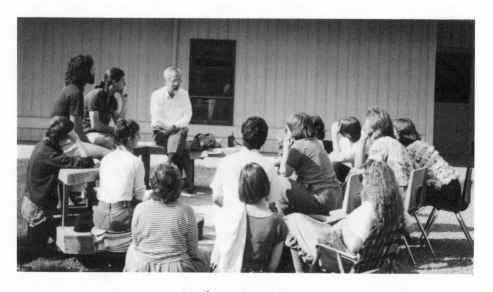

Student Questions

Q: I would like to ask you about Taoist philosophy. You said there was not much to speak about, yet you teach it, so there must be something you could say.

Master Ni: What I teach is not Taoism, but the true spiritual achievement of the ancients. Harmony and balance are the basic principles of life. Beyond that, what else can be said? Not much. The most important thing is whether we can achieve normalcy in our lives. Are our minds aligned with the *t'ai chi* principle at each moment? What besides this can be called the Way?

The Way is not something outside of us that we can pursue or worship. We need to realize the *t'ai chi* principle of harmony and balance in our daily lives. The Way is not a conceptual activity. It is life itself, in its totality. We are all the offspring of nature, and each of us is a small model of nature. To be the Way is more important than talking about what the Way is.

We are naturally born as a *t'ai chi*, but after experiencing worldly life, we are affected by our surroundings. We need to examine how well we handle the effects of life around us. If we become upset when we cannot achieve something or if we are bothered by someone who has a bad attitude toward us or who does not play fair, how are we to respond? In *T'ai Chi* movement, we learn not to fight but to yield. If people attack you, a gentle movement can transform the situation. A *t'ai chi* can always move around. If you allow yourself to move, the attack remains only a situation and does not escalate into something more.

On the other hand, it may not be someone else who is bothering you. Maybe the real problem is that you are not conscious enough and are therefore bothering someone else. In that case, you need to immediately correct yourself. In any situation, we must move just right: not too much, not too little. If we move too little, friction or conflict comes. If we move too much, we exhaust ourselves and are trapped.

We cannot leave the world to seek peace. There is no peace in life. There is no total security. If you think you need security, stand right here where you are and do *T'ai Chi* movement. It will protect you and not damage anyone else. I believe all of you are wise enough to move without creating problems, but sometimes you need to watch your emotions, especially toward yourself. You say, "Damn this, damn that," and become really unhappy. Allow yourself to move around with *T'ai Chi* movement. If you move too far in one direction, you have nowhere to go and have to turn around. This is important to remember.

Some of you may think that a spiritual life consists of meditating all day long. That is not the Way, that is a dead end. The real practitioner of the Way keeps moving. We enjoy our lives and enjoy *t'ai chi*. *T'ai chi* is accomplished through our lives. Each moment is a self-accomplishing completeness.

You might ask me, "Master Ni, how can you describe movement without talking about stillness?" Do you really think that there is no movement in stillness? Even when you do not move, you are still moving, but the movement is subtle. You are breathing and thinking; strongly or gently, you are doing something. If you do not keep moving, your body will deteriorate. Life itself is movement.

Our destiny in each moment is to move correctly and sustain the natural flow of life within us. Maybe you think you need to surpass your destiny by going to a mountain where you can stop moving and breathing and fossilize yourself, but is that really surpassing life? Life and nature are constantly living, moving, working and generating. Once we stop generating, we degenerate.

Each cell of your body is a *t'ai chi*. We are each a small model of the universe, thus we are each a small but complete *t'ai chi*. Inside, we are composed of even smaller *t'ai chi's* that need us to keep moving. An even temper, pleasant nature, healthful life, youthful appearance, and everything fine about you, all come from good movement. The Way includes both movement and stillness. It is from stillness that we learn to move. Many years ago, we were stones.

Q: How is the practice of T'ai Chi Chuan *related to spiritual self-cultivation?*

Master Ni: Although *T'ai Chi Chuan* is considered by some to be a martial art, it is not really involved with fighting. It is actually the practice of ancient cosmology. Through the practice of *T'ai Chi* Movement, the universal spirit may exhibit itself, both inside and outside of the body, so that one may unite with it. It is a necessary cultivation.

Let me give you a practical illustration. What a person learns, and the kind of activities he or she engages in, influence the personality. A person who studies and practices martial arts with the fighting aspect in mind tends to be more inclined toward fighting, has less self-control and is hot-tempered. *T'ai Chi* movements are a method of balancing oneself physically, emotionally and spiritually. Gentle physical arts are a self-healing practice which can be done every day by anyone of any age in any physical condition. My *T'ai Chi* exercise is different from ordinary *T'ai Chi Chuan*, because it implements the principles contained in Lao Tzu's *Tao Teh Ching* (or the *Way of Life*) and the *Book of Changes and the Unchanging Truth*.

I do not teach martial arts, but I sometimes mention the application of the *t'ai chi* principle in practicing them, because a physical illustration can help someone understand it better. I learned *T'ai Chi* exercise as part of the ancient spiritual tradition, but not for fighting purposes. It is certainly an effective method of self-defense, but its essential value is that of a philosophical and spiritual practice.

Q: Would you say more about the emotions and how to balance them?

Master Ni: Because we live in a commercialized culture, we are constantly being stimulated by what look like beautiful events. Mass advertising creates beliefs or expectations in people's minds. Then, when life does not match their expectations, undeveloped people cannot handle their disappointment well, and they react emotionally.

Most people are emotional yo-yos. They go up and down, up and down, sometimes really excited, then later feeling terrible. You need to watch yourself in everyday life. There is a basic line to life. It is not a line which moves up and down. The basic line is the point where you are feeling just plain comfortable or all right. The *T'ai Chi* practitioner always looks for that base line. Once you find the base line, and learn to stay near it, your life will be smoother, because you will not allow your energy flow to go too high and pass over the base line. You also will not allow your emotions to sink too far below it.

You must learn to accept the fact that emotions come, and then they leave. Emotions are related to the internal chemistry of the body. Try to discover what stimulates your emotions in repetitive patterns, and then avoid those things or learn to accept them with a different mind set or attitude. This can minimize their effect or help you use them constructively. It is important to understand yourself, including your emotions. This is true of both men and women. Morning and night, your moods differ because your energy level is different. Sometimes you are affected by the sun cycle, and sometimes by the moon cycle. Your home and work environments also affect you and can cause disharmony unless you learn to manage them.

One way to do this is to get up earlier. If you continue to sleep after the sun has risen, your energy will be congested in your head. *T'ai Chi* movement, or any gentle movement, can take the congestion away, but we will talk about that later. Getting up earlier is the first way to improve your life.

People sometimes spoil themselves by thinking, "I am an adult, and I can do whatever I like." Yes, you surely can, but it will not make you happy. Even being too excited can make your energy explode and sometimes cause unhappiness. You cannot see this kind of explosion with your eyes, but it happens internally. Afterwards, it is hard to gather yourself back in one piece. If you are not in one piece, then how can you expect to have a smooth emotional flow?

Some women, especially during menstruation or ovulation, become nervous and irritable and feel like crying when their energy is pulled down to the abdomen. Some do cry, because of the low cycle. It is usually easy to manage the high cycle, because you feel happy and life is enjoyable, but it is often hard to manage the low cycle. During low cycles I suggest that you not move, not think, and not make any decisions or judgments. Anything you do in a low cycle can result in an emotional explosion. You will hate yourself if you say something unkind to your boyfriend or to a good friend when your emotions are low. If you stay quiet, you do not need to ask people to forgive you afterward.

Because modern life is so fast paced, some of you have a hard time gathering yourself into one piece. Modern people do not live better than ancient people who lived a simple life. You have more material goods, but you are so rushed and scattered that your enjoyment or relaxation is less. In modern times, you have to choose: will you swim fast like a small fish on the surface of the water, or will you glide slowly through deeper pools? Truthfully, you do not need much influence from society. Accept only as much as you can take. If it is too much, do not push yourself further. Give yourself a retreat.

Q: Generally speaking, Westerners have been raised differently from the people of the East and therefore have a much different mental structure. With this in mind, is it possible for Westerners to truly absorb and digest the teachings of the East?

Master Ni: All human beings have the same true nature. All differences are cultural, and all cultures distort people's minds. If you thoroughly understand the nature of culture, you know that it is just like a suit of clothes.

For instance, I come from China. I can wear Chinese clothes and look like a Chinaman, but I can also wear Western clothes. I do not emphasize cultural differences. They are simply historical accumulations that can create confusion and cause people to lose sight of their true nature. If your mind is open and unprejudiced, then your spirit is high. If you have Western antiques with Oriental decorations in your house, and you feel it all fits, that's fine. Nothing fights anything else, because your high spirit is in a position to enjoy all of it. If any culture or religion makes you feel confused or troubled, it is an unnecessary and unhealthy hindrance and obstacle.

After you recognize and respect your true nature, then you can enjoy the benefits of all cultures. If you let world cultures confuse you, they cease to be a tonic and become a poison that needs to be eliminated from your mind. Many people cannot make good use of their cultures. They blindly emphasize the differences or the specialness of one particular culture, making the world even more confused. This is a human defect that is not consistent with high spiritual understanding.

Q: Do you do other exercises besides T'ai Chi *movement?*

Master Ni: *T'ai Chi* is also a principle, so there are different movements and different practices. You can do *T'ai Chi* standing, sitting or lying down. You can also visualize yourself doing it. In the morning, I do a type of sitting *T'ai Chi* called *Dao-In*. There are different types of *T'ai Chi* movements that are used according to the situation.

I usually talk about internal *T'ai Chi* as being more important than external *T'ai Chi*. The goal is obviously the same, to attain harmony and balance. Without practicing internal *T'ai Chi*, external *T'ai Chi* only reminds your mind to attune yourself. Internal *T'ai*

Chi is a system that goes beneath or beyond external form. That is the key.

So to answer your question, do I do anything besides *T'ai Chi?* Yes, I do lots of things. There is an abundance of ancient methods that were developed through millions of years of human experience. Few people have the time to learn them all, but at least you know *T'ai Chi.*

Many people think, "I like living in this body, but I would also like to prove that my life extends beyond this physical life." You can use *T'ai Chi* movement to prove this for yourself. I do that practice also: at the beginning I do it intentionally with my mind. When I am asleep, my soul can stand up, walk outdoors and practice *T'ai Chi* from beginning to end and then come back. Usually, if you do one or two movements, it is an astral projection. After you do those one or two movements, you lose yourself and are already asleep again. It is quite difficult to do the whole sequence through, but it is worth a try. It must happen in real sleep. If you use the mind, you will suddenly wake up, because the mind and the soul are different.

Once you have enough training and have practiced persistently, any movement you make can connect your body, mind and spirit. Even if you only think the words, "*T'ai Chi,*" you will immediately align yourself in one piece. How do you do it? By deep practice. There is a Chinese proverb that says, "When you learn to do movement, keep doing the movement at all times. When you learn to sing, keep singing until you sing well." This means, when you learn *T'ai Chi* movement, move your body as if you were doing *T'ai Chi* movement at all times. When you learn dancing, move as if you were dancing all the time. This is how you achieve yourself.

There are many spiritual treasures to be learned. Don't feel disappointed if you do not have enough time to learn them all. We are fortunate enough to learn *T'ai Chi. T'ai Chi* opens the door to high achievement, and I hope all of you will have the chance to learn it.

When I was young, I traveled to the high mountains to visit many masters. I will tell you the truth: many of them did not know *T'ai Chi* at all! Then how did they live so long and achieve so highly? Each of them knew some simple movement that had a specific benefit. You have already learned much more than any master, but you must practice it. Constancy and persistence are the keys to success. You will learn many things as you continue to practice *chi* movement and implement the *t'ai chi* principle in your everyday life.

When chi flows smoothly,
you are healthy.
When sen (spirit) is clear,
you are happy
when nothing happens!

气畅左不悖

神舒在不为

化情

Chapter 2

Choosing the Exercise that is Right for You

There are different ways to maintain the form of life.
Students of life nurture the subtle essence.
Students of death only excite the body.
A balanced life comes from caring for both the body
*   and the essence.*   - Lao Tzu

Section 1: Comparing the Different Types

I

Exercises Have Different Purposes

Master Ni: Each *chi* movement has a special purpose. When you understand the function of each movement, then you can choose the one that is right for you. All the different styles I teach can help you develop yourself. There are three sets of *T'ai Chi* movement called Gentle Path, Sky Journey and Infinite Expansion, and another type of gentle movement called Cosmic Tour *Ba Gua Zahn*. *Dao-In* is unique in its own scope.

The Eight Treasures, Harmony/Trinity *T'ai Chi* and Self-Healing *Chi Gong* are available on videotape by Dr. Maoshing Ni. Crane Style *Chi Gong* is available on videotape, with an accompanying book, by Dr. Daoshing Ni. Learning from videotapes or attending classes will enhance one's health and refine one's spirit.

Many kinds of therapeutic *Chi Kung* (or *Chi Gong*) have been developed and reorganized by teachers in mainland China. Dr. Daoshing Ni chose White Crane Style for its simplicity and helpfulness. It is not an ancient method, but it has proven useful to beginners in mainland China and overseas.

Generally speaking, I recommend that you learn the Eight Treasures first, then the Harmony/Trinity *T'ai Chi*, which is a simplified form of Gentle Path. Then learn Gentle Path, Sky Journey, and Infinite Expansion. You can practice all of them according to different seasons, different times of day and as a preparation for various activities. The greatest knowledge and awareness come from experiencing all the exercises and understanding your internal situation.

Dao-In, Chi Kung (Chi Gong), the Six Healing Sounds[2] and other practices are all useful on specific occasions. Find the practice you like best and stick with it, but remain flexible, because on

---

[2]This practice is described in the books *Awaken to the Great Path* (originally published as *Uncharted Voyage Toward the Subtle Light*) and *Power of Natural Healing*.

27

certain occasions you may prefer to do something else. Knowing a variety or variation of movements can help you avoid a monotonous or uninteresting practice.

There are many valuable things to learn. What you learn depends upon your stage of growth and your level of development. In order to make room for new things, sometimes you have to give up some old things. We are always in the process of learning something better and giving up something less important. What was very important at an early stage will eventually become less important. This is general guidance for how to choose a suitable movement.

Next I will make a broad comparison between different types of movement. Then I will give suggestions for how to select a practice that is right for you. In Chapter Three, I will discuss the individual forms in greater detail.

II
Chi Kung (*Chi Gong*) and *T'ai Chi* Movement

Chi Kung (*Chi Gong*) is a general name for all kinds of gentle movement, both internal and external, that directly activate or help guide a smooth flow of *chi* throughout the body by use of the breath, simple movements, posture, and mental imagery. By releasing tension and stimulating vitality, the practice of *Chi Kung* (*Chi Gong*) promotes self-healing and strengthens the immune system. Some forms are a complete set of different movements, while others are just one or more simple movements. Each movement has a different effect.

T'ai Chi is a specific type of *Chi Kung* (*Chi Gong*) practice. In general, *Chi Kung* (Chi *Gong*) is usually much simpler than *T'ai Chi*. *T'ai Chi* consists of many *Chi Kung* (Chi Gong) movements that are arranged according to the principles of the *Tao Teh Ching* and the *I Ching*[3]. Different levels of practice all come from this common foundation.

Chi Kung (*Chi Gong*)

Master Ni: *Chi Kung* (*Chi Gong)* has many different levels. I will describe three of them here. The first level is for someone with a

---

[3]Also called *The Book of Changes*.

physical problem, such as an injured or diseased organ or body part. This is called Healing *Chi Kung* (*Chi Gong*). The second level is for preventive purposes and to enhance the vital force (life strength) internally and externally. This is called *Dao-In* or *chi* practice.

In ancient times, the third level was not called *Chi Kung* (*Chi Gong*); it was called spiritual practice. However, a good spiritual practice is directly connected with energy transformation and management, so it can be called *Chi Kung* (*Chi Gong*) too. Any practice that takes place on the subtle rather than the visible level, such as developing a good mind, inspiring wisdom, increasing memory power, increasing spiritual power or uplifting oneself to a different level of immortality can be called *Chi Kung* (*Chi Gong*).

Everyone can benefit from learning some kind of *Chi Kung* (*Chi Gong*): standing *Chi Kung* (*Chi Gong*), sitting *Chi Kung* (*Chi Gong*), sleeping *Chi Kung* (*Chi Gong*), etc. *Chi Kung* (*Chi Gong*) is a tool for building health and for taking responsibility for your whole life, internally and externally.

T'ai Chi Movement

Master Ni: Like *Chi Kung* (*Chi Gong*), *T'ai Chi* movement also has many levels. As you practice over the years, your experience changes. Your interest and energy manifestation are also different.

T'ai Chi is a series of harmonized movements governed by cosmic principles. Because a *t'ai chi* is whole, the movements are connected like flowing water. You cannot divide them into separate parts.

As in handwriting, each individual expresses his or her own personality when practicing *T'ai Chi*. *T'ai Chi* for personal development is always adaptable to personal differences and stages of individual development.

III
Movement is Like Water

Master Ni: The variation between each of the internal arts is like the difference between swimming in a lake, a river or an ocean. Each gives you a different experience, according to their distinct currents and flows. By experiencing their variations, you deepen and widen yourself.

Spiritually, you may need to know only one leaf to know the whole tree, or one spoonful of water to know the whole ocean. Realistically, however, it can take years of training to know the whole tree or the ocean, but not by looking at the leaves or the water.

You can compare the three types of *T'ai Chi* Exercise to water. If you follow the recommended course of learning, first you experience Gentle Path movement, which is like the water in a lake or canal, so peaceful it is almost still. Then you experience Sky Journey, whose movements are like the water of a river. The third movement, Infinite Expansion, is like the water of the ocean. An ocean can have many whirlpools, but the movements of Infinite Expansion do not make you dizzy, because they consist of natural energy.

Modern people enjoy surfing waves, but gentle physical movement is a kind of internal energy surfing. You can enjoy this kind of surfing without having to buy any expensive equipment. Also, you do not need to worry about arthritis from exposure to water, wind or cold, or that your bones will suffer from other trouble. All forms of *T'ai Chi* movement are trouble-free energy surfing. *T'ai Chi* practice should never be forced or stiff like a military drill.

IV

Organized and Controlled Approach
vs. Creative and Flexible Approach

Master Ni: Although to the untrained eye they may look similar, the styles of gentle physical arts are not the same. For example, Cosmic Tour *Ba Gua Zahn* is not like eating a meal that is already prepared. Cosmic Tour is almost like going into the kitchen and creating a new dish for yourself. You can do part of it or the whole thing, and you can start with any one of the movements. You can make it simple or complicated, and you can do it quickly or slowly, because you are the cook.

Yet, when you do Gentle Path, Sky Journey or Infinite Expansion *T'ai Chi*, generations of practitioners have made the sequence from one movement to the next more tightly linked and thus more controlled. Surely, after learning the movements, you can make some variation by changing some movements from left to right, right to left, backward to forward, forward to backward, and so forth. However, because each movement has an important function within the context of the whole form, they are not as free or adjustable as Cosmic Tour or the Eight Treasures.

V
Each Exercise Focuses on a Center

Master Ni: Each type of movement usually has a focal point or center that brings a specific benefit. By knowing that center and by understanding the function of each movement, the benefit is usually greater. Let us discuss the *tan tien*, which are the three main energy centers of the body.

A *tan tien* is an internal energy center located in a specific region of the body. In modern terms, it could be called a nerve center. Many parts of the body can be a specific energy field. Thus, you can consider a *tan tien* to be everywhere, particularly in a person who is achieved and is able to gather energy anywhere he or she desires.

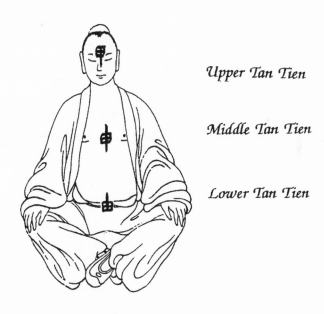

Upper Tan Tien

Middle Tan Tien

Lower Tan Tien

The Three *Tan Tien*

There are three *Tan Tien* in the human body. The Upper *Tan Tien* is located inside the central point between the eyebrows.

The Middle *Tan Tien* is located inside the central point of the chest. The Lower *Tan Tien* is inside the lower abdomen. When the concentration is focused on one of these areas, different effects are produced.

Gentle Path Movement, which is centered in the Lower *Tan Tien*, is sometimes called Peace on Earth. Sky Journey, which is centered in the Middle *Tan Tien,* is sometimes called Harmony with People. Infinite Expansion, which is centered in the axis of the upright trunk of the body, is sometimes called Uniting with Heaven. The axis, which runs from the perineum to the midpoint at the top of the head, goes through all three *Tan Tien*.

The Eight Treasures and *Dao-In* were originally the same exercise, with different applications. Both are designed to attune your internal energy, including circulation and glandular secretions, stimulation and generation, thereby preventing and removing stagnation and blockage. They harmonize and strengthen the body naturally, without focusing on a specific energy center or *Tan Tien*.

You might have seen some pictures of famous *T'ai Chi* teachers. Teachers who over-emphasize the Lower *Tan Tien* become plump, with a thick waist. I do not think plumpness is very good, from the standpoint of health, so please practice several other types of gentle movements as well. Eating or sleeping too much will also cause you to have a big waist.

VI

Functions of the Movements

Master Ni: Different kinds of movement are valued for different reasons. For example, Gentle Path *T'ai Chi* movement builds up your energy or *chi*. Sky Journey motivates you to move gracefully. Infinite Expansion trains you to be naturally in perfect control of your body and physical energy. It is a good exercise, but it is a little stronger than Sky Journey and Gentle Path.

T'ai Chi movement has become more popular than *Ba Gua Zahn* or Cosmic Tour among the last generation of scholars. The movements are still equally valuable in building health, which is to say, they have a similar healing power as *T'ai Chi*, but the energy flow is different.

Chi Kung (Chi Gong) is for health. *Dao-In* and Eight Treasures are for longevity. Push hands and martial arts are for practical purposes of competition. Sword practice is for spiritual concentration and total integration. Please see Chapter 3 for specific details about each type of movement.

Section 2: Specific Guidance For Selecting a Practice

Master Ni: In selecting a practice, you need to consider the stage of life you are in and your physical condition. I recommend that you read this entire book before making your choice.

Q: Can't I just pick any type of movement and learn it?

Master Ni: Certainly, but you would benefit even more by making an informed selection. *Chi Kung (Chi Gong)* is typically a gentle movement that is combined with the practice of breathing, and most types of *Chi Kung (Chi Gong)* are suitable for most people.

When you have a physical problem or illness, you need to consider what kind of exercise is appropriate for you. Please see the section below on People with Special Health Considerations.

Vigorous kinds of *Chi Kung (Chi Gong)* are only suitable for people who are very healthy and strong. These styles are popular because of their quickly noticeable effects. That is the positive side. The negative aspect is that these forms tend to lead you away from your original purpose.

When you are too physical, any kind of gentle movement can be a spiritual discipline to help you attain better self-control.

Children

Master Ni: I do not recommend that children learn any *chi* practice before they are eight years old. They should be allowed to be natural and do what they like within reason. Some parents who have a martial arts or *Chi Kung (Chi Gong)* foundation push their children into it, but that is not a good idea. It is better to allow children to be natural. They can learn when they are older.

After about the age of 10, a child's energy needs to be channelled or trained. At that time it is suitable for them to learn a martial art, or *Chi Kung (Chi Gong)* or *T'ai Chi*. Usually *T'ai Chi* training is a little too complicated for beginners, so simple martial arts are good for them and can also help their self-confidence.

Q: What kind of exercise is best for an 8 or 10 year old?

Master Ni: I can only speak generally, because each child is different. Because the Eight Treasures is such a good foundation for all other types of gentle movement, if they learn that first, then in later years they can learn whatever they wish. Children might also enjoy the simplified version of Cosmic Tour *Ba Gua Zahn* called Merry-Go-Round.

When I was young, people thought I was from Northern China, because the people from the South are usually short. The reason I was tall was from doing the Eight Treasures. Teenagers who are afraid of being too short will have good results from learning the Eight Treasures.

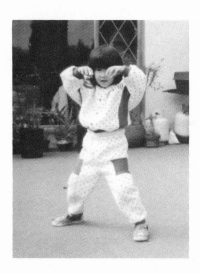

Q: Should young people join an adult exercise class, or are there special classes for children?

Master Ni: I think that young children can join adult classes if the adults are learning a simple kind of movement. When youngsters join an adult class, the teachers usually do not need to give specific attention or discipline to the youngsters, they will naturally try to follow well.

I personally do not have any specific experience with teaching youngsters, because in my classes I prefer a combination of all ages and both sexes. However, someone suggested that I have a martial arts summer camp for children. That is a good idea. I wish that more active teachers would try this type of activity, because it could increase the popularity of the physical arts and also serve the young generation.

Q: Is there a good way for parents to help their children exercise more or become more interested in exercise?

Master Ni: The best help is keep the television turned off in the early morning and evening. Also, when parents exercise, the children are sometimes inspired to follow and learn. Parents need to encourage them, but not push them to do it.

When Dao and Mao were young, I occasionally brought them to my classes. As they became friends with the adults and younger students in the class, they were naturally encouraged to learn without my specific attention.

Q: Is there anything else you wish to say about children?

Master Ni: Parents need to pay attention to the normal growth of their children. It is important that they not develop negative habits, like a fondness for one kind of food or for soft drinks, which are bad for health. If the environment includes different physical activities, that will naturally guide the children. For example, if there is a pole in the house, a child will naturally learn to climb the pole, etc. That is a healthy child.

Children need the freedom to explore all healthy directions. A society or a family should have a good library. They also can offer good opportunities for children to develop any healthy interest that will benefit their growth.

My personal development was well established by the time I was a teenager. I had learned calligraphy, reading, writing, internal martial arts, meditation, Chinese medicine, different systems of divination, spiritual practice, and so forth. Those things were my hobbies when I was young. Finally I became proficient in them. It took years to accomplish, but the early years laid the foundation. It is important for young people to have the opportunity and freedom to explore all kinds of healthy hobbies and interests for their future development.

Young People

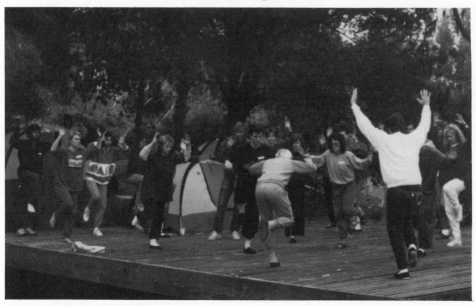

Master Ni: Young people who have a lot of time and energy might like to learn all the movements I have taught. A young person whose goal is to know himself or herself through gentle physical exercise or martial arts will benefit greatly by learning a variety of skills.

Q: If someone wants to learn several forms, how many hours a day should they practice? How many forms can they learn at once?

Master Ni: That is an interesting question. It takes some time to learn any form well. In China, some people have learned so many forms that it would take about ten minutes just to recite them. That is a type of ambition and an interesting exploration, but that kind of expansion proves nothing in particular. It is best to start with one form and learn it well before adding any others.

Q: If a person is learning and practicing diligently, should they limit their practice to a certain number of hours each day?

Master Ni: No, I do not think there should be a limitation, because practice is how people achieve themselves. If somebody achieves less, it is because the interest is different. The amount of time you spend practicing is an individual matter; you should learn and practice according to your own opportunities and needs.

I do not approve of families who shut their young sons or daughters in the garden and make them practice *T'ai Chi* for eight or ten hours a day. I have heard that some members of the Chen family do 20 to 40 repetitions of the same simple formula. With that kind of fervor, they may achieve a certain level in fighting, but I have never heard that anyone in the Chen family has ever lived to be a hundred years old.

Q: Is there a certain way you feel when you have done enough or too much?

Master Ni: Each person has their own natural internal clock. You know how long is right for you. I do it rhythmically. That means sometimes I do one form, stop, and then do another form. Sometimes I exercise for 20 minutes with music, then sometimes I continue with no music.

The main principle in whatever you do is to do it for enjoyment, not for external reasons. If you force yourself to do it, it will bring no benefit. If you do it for enjoyment, then you become a *shien*, which is a happy spiritual individual. That is the goal. Enjoyment comes from avoiding suffering. Do not create suffering for yourself by letting your mind betray your kingdom of life.

Middle-Aged People

Q: As a middle aged person, I do not have as much endurance or energy as I used to. Which exercise would be most suitable for me to learn?

Master Ni: Middle age is a golden time, for both men and women. When you are young, you look beautiful no matter what you wear, but in middle age, you have to watch your grooming more carefully. Similarly, if you do not work on your body during this time, you cannot expect to have a healthy old age. In middle age, although business and career are important, all areas of personal life such as body, mind and spirit need to have good exercise if you wish to have a long happy life.

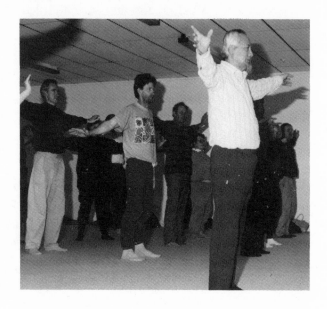

Middle-aged people can start with the Eight Treasures; either the simple form or the complete form is good for them. The simple form is often taught by general teachers. It is sometimes called the "Eight Pieces of Embroidery" and is simply the first movement of each section of the Eight Treasures, without the internal movement.

Middle-aged people are usually family people, although some are single. If you learn *Chi Kung (Chi Gong)* in middle-age, you can easily see the progress or attainment from your practice. For example, you can tolerate long work hours better, have more sexual stamina, and so forth.

On the one hand, you need to build up your energy during middle age, but you also need to be disciplined, because like a flower or a fruit tree, you have reached your peak, so you should be conservative with your energy. Ancient philosophy reminds us that when the moon becomes full, it will soon wane. When a flower is fully opened, it is about to fade. This is why, at the high point of your life, you need to be more careful and restrain yourself to make the good time last longer.

Before 30 you are young; after 40 you are middle-aged. With proper practice and self-care, you can prolong your middle age from 40 to 80. Then from 80 to 120 you can consider yourself a mature person. You should be young at heart, but you need to restrain yourself from going to extremes or indulging in extravagances during your middle age.

Older People

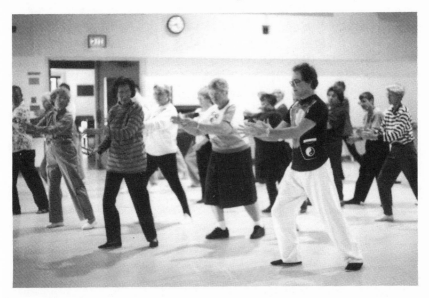

Q: Would you talk about chi *exercise for older people?*

Master Ni: I do not like the word old. The number of years one has lived does not describe one's condition. Weakness or sickness can happen to people of any age. People in later life can also be healthy and strong. Many people accept the concept of age and eventually allow that concept to destroy or reduce their health.

If you overuse yourself and burn out like a candle, how can you bring new energy into yourself? The prevention of aging and discovering methods of rejuvenation are both the focus of the science of the Integral Way. *Chi Kung (Chi Gong)* practice through gentle movement is good for helping you recover from an exhausting career.

First you need to dissolve your preconceptions about age. In the morning, the sunshine is fresh and great. At noon, the sunshine is brightest, but in the evening it is the most beautiful. Value your evening years by extending your health, your mental faculties, and your subtle life on the spiritual level. Your soul can achieve great progress that will prepare it for transformation and higher evolution.

Q: Which exercise should older people start with?

Master Ni: I suggest some form of *Chi Kung* (*Chi Gong*) such as Eight Treasures. *Dao-In* may be more suitable, because it can be done in a sitting position. Some *Dao-In* movements are difficult, but most of them can be done easily in a sitting or lying position. Seated *Dao-In* is more suitable for a mature person to practice; a vigorous individual whose emotions are not suited to this gentle exercise might not enjoy it. There are many systems that can be practiced if you wish to become rougher, but I suggest that you become gentler.

People who are physically weak or aging fast would greatly benefit from doing Gentle Path *T'ai Chi*. When you are older, you have less vitality. Exercise increases vitality, and the value of Gentle Path is rejuvenation.

As people age, they usually notice weakness in their legs. Aging also causes one's energy to float up to the head, which can cause high blood pressure or a stroke. Cosmic Tour can fight problems of aging by bringing energy back down into the legs. It can also make the bones and the whole body very flexible. Older people who wish to learn it can start by walking in a short, straight line, back and forth, then in a bigger circle, then adding hand, body and leg postures to channel the energy. Do not force anything or overextend yourself. Take it easy and build up your strength gradually.

Q: In China, aren't there many older people who practice T'ai Chi *every morning in the parks?*

Master Ni: Yes, there are, and I encourage my friends to offer such a service in this country as well. Usually there is no charge for such a class, it is a pure service. Some of my students charge $1 for each class.

Dr. Maoshing Ni: Gentle *Chi Kung (Chi Gong)* or *T'ai Chi* are not like the cardio-vascular aerobic exercises that are popular in technologically advanced societies. People in China, who regularly practice gentle movement, live to be 80 or 90 without ever developing heart disease or high blood pressure or other age related diseases that are common in the United States. Millions of Chinese people go out every morning at 5 a.m. to do *chi* exercises. Some of them are quite advanced in age, yet they still have vitality and exuberance because their *chi* is strong. Everyone has the potential to master their own body and their own *chi* by cultivating themselves and thus preventing the decline in health that happens to so many older people.

Q: If someone is 50 years old and has never exercised much in their life, is it dangerous for them to start?

Master Ni: First of all, 50 years is not very old, it is still young, and a young person has the potential to learn anything that is suitable. They need to start slowly and gently, and practice regularly.

Q: What about someone in their 60s, 70s, and 80s? Can they still start to exercise at that age?

Master Ni: Definitely. That is middle-age. They should simply proceed slowly and gently.

Many people die in middle age; I mean before 80. That is a pity, because they could have learned something that would have made them more physically independent than relying on medication or a doctor and abandoning their natural potential for a long and happy life.

Q: Is there anything that older people need to be careful about when they do T'ai Chi practice, or any kind of Eight Treasures or Dao-In?

Master Ni: The school of internal harmony usually teaches gentle movement, so a trained teacher or trained individual knows to go in gradual steps rather than big leaps.

Q: How long should an older person practice every day?

Master Ni: It is not a matter of age, but of how much the exercise affects them. If someone walks one mile he might be tired, but another person might walk a couple of miles and still be fresh. It depends on the individual.

When you start exercising, stop before you feel exhausted. A little tiredness is okay, such as when you climb a steep slope and begin to pant. Just do not over exert yourself. Gradually build yourself up through gentle movement. Be relaxed when you do it. Tension is what kills you, not gentle, graceful movements.

Q: Is there a certain age at which people should stop doing T'ai Chi *movement?*

Master Ni: *T'ai Chi*, at a higher and deeper level, is not a form. Whenever you walk or do a small chore or housework, by alternately moving both legs or both hands up and down, left and right, first one and then the other, you are doing *T'ai Chi*. The *t'ai chi* principle encompasses life itself. When your life stops, there is no more *t'ai chi*. You cannot rely on the narrow sense of the *T'ai Chi* form alone. If you are superstitious and think that *T'ai Chi* can make you live forever, you are dreaming. What you can rely on is your internal life, all your vital forces.

You need to know one other thing. Life and death are natural, alternate stages of life. Death is not about death; death is about a new life; so do not be afraid of it. If you are afraid of death, and you keep doing *T'ai Chi*, you will be using it to condition your consciousness to go deeper into your fear. Life is for enjoyment, for growth. Whatever you enjoy, like *Nei Kung* (internal work) and *Chi Kung* (*Chi Gong*) (physical movement with breathing technique) are all helpful and useful when you master them. *Nei Kung* is the internal rather than external movement of energy. Internal and external movements united are *Chi Kung (Chi Gong)*.

If you are going to die, and you know that physically and internally everything is all right, you will have a natural death. If you wish to postpone your death, practice holding your breath, then the internal pressure will be increased. If you repeatedly practice this every day, your vitality will recover. There are many other methods for regeneration and revitalization. This is the whole subject of the Integral Way.

Q: If an older person practices Chi Kung *and meditation, exactly what kind of rejuvenation can they expect?*

Master Ni: Better health, better physique and better mental function.

I do not recommend this, but sometimes I test myself to see how old I am. I went to Magic Mountain and Disneyland and sat on the roller coaster with some youngsters for the 360-degree circle. I found out that I am the same as a young child. I have tried many things to see if I can do what they can do, but I do not encourage everyone to do that.

What I recommend in my books is my personal experience, not an empty replication of someone else's system. My subjective and objective evaluation allows me to make a conservative estimate that if a person follows what I describe in my books, they can lengthen their life and health for at least 20 to 30 years. Of course greater achievement is still possible, depending on the individual.

Q: Can a person become physically strong again?

Master Ni: What you can do is slow down your aging so that you age at the speed of a turtle instead of a rabbit. You slow the aging process, but you do not slow down your good mind. In the last 20 years, I have accomplished many things. I do not think there are many young people who can write six books a year or travel tens of thousands of miles a year like I do. They are too young.

Q: Can older people do chi *practice for the purpose of spiritual cultivation?*

Master Ni: Certainly, if they do it as a natural spiritual discipline. If they talk about spiritual cultivation and immediately feel tight or stiff like a religious set-up, it will be of no help. Having natural spiritual confidence is a key to one's later years. With natural spiritual confidence, people's vitality becomes stronger as they grow older. It is important for everyone to develop the natural endowment that is within each person and to work on any areas in which they feel insufficient. Nature does not limit a person's development, only a conditioned mind can do that.

Men

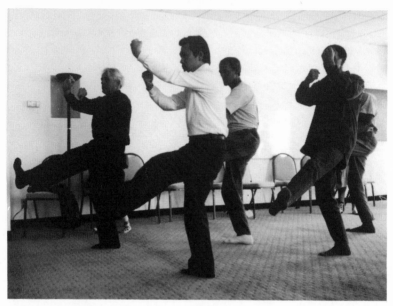

Q: Do you have any specific advice for men?

Master Ni: When it comes to practicing *T'ai Chi* movement, I think men and women are almost the same.

In my tradition, a person's sexual health is very important. Even if you are not sexually active, you can still maintain internal sexual health. Although you may have the same impulse as a sixteen year old, you have much better control, because you know that the root of your longevity comes from this source. I have written other books about this topic, specifically *Harmony: The Art of Life*.

Q: Does a construction worker or mechanic need to do this kind of exercise?

Master Ni: No. Physical workers need emotional and mental

relaxation more than physical movement. What the internal school teaches is totally different from muscular work. Physical work cannot attune and strengthen you in the same balanced way that gentle movement can.

Q: Is there any particular exercise that celibate men should do?

Master Ni: In general, celibacy is of no use. Both men and women have sexual dreams if they are celibate. If you do not use that muscle, it will become useless. These practices can help you maintain complete health. Although there are certain practices specifically for sexual health, they are not the focus of this book, which is how to choose an exercise that makes you completely healthy.

The body is like a generator of electric energy, but it is also like a battery that stores energy. The top of the head is the positive end of the battery, and the bottom of the body, at the perineum, is the negative end. You always need to recharge yourself through internal movement and from natural energy sources: the earth, sun, moon, and stars all support you.

All of the exercises presented in this book are suitable for either celibate or sexually active men. Their main focus is health. They will make you strong and make your *chi* strong, but if you use that *chi* for sexual fantasies, there is no benefit in that.

Q: You have said that cultivation should not be done three days before and four days after sex. What if somebody is very active sexually, say two times a week? Can they not learn any of these exercises?

Master Ni: I do not think there are many people who can follow those guidelines very well. *T'ai Chi* teachers who don't follow the regulation may achieve more power than other people, but they will have shorter lives.

Women

Q: Which exercises are especially good for women?

Master Ni: As I said, I think that women and men are not very different in this respect. Some women are more athletic than others.

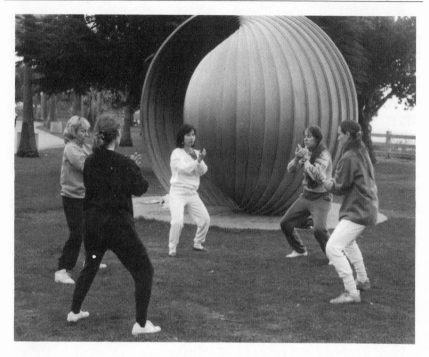

I have learned from women teachers, too, and many arts were developed by women teachers. So almost everything I teach is suitable for women.

Q: Should a woman exercise during her menstrual period?

Master Ni: No. It is not suitable for a woman who practices cultivation. Today, women use tampons so they can jog and engage in other rough physical activities, but I think that is damaging. I think that during menstruation a woman should let nature take its course and not create any external interference.

Q: So even if a woman uses pads, she should not do chi *exercise during her period?*

Master Ni: She can do general everyday activities, but no vigorous movement. A few *Chi Kung* (*Chi Gong*) movements can be done at any time, including menstruation; ask your instructor.

Q: What should a woman do for spiritual purposes?

Master Ni: For women, the Golden Medicine is refined before sexual arousal each midnight. Before menstruation, you gather the pure energy and let the impure energy go. When you sit in meditation at this time, gently draw the pure energy up to the higher centers so that it can enhance the soul.[4]

During menstruation, do not allow the *chi* to flow down and out of the body. Let go of the visible things, like the blood and the lining of the uterus. The practice of Golden Medicine does not deal with substantial things, the Golden Medicine is the insubstantial *chi* you have gathered to nurture yourself.

This is not to say you should not meditate during menstruation. I am simply suggesting that you be sure to meditate before it starts. In general, if you consistently meditate every day, particularly before your period begins, you may be able reduce the heavy outflow of energy. Actually, after you have taken the pure energy, it does not even matter if you have a heavy flow, if what flows is merely physical.

Q: Should a pregnant woman do chi *exercise?*

Master Ni: Some gentle movements are all right. Some women, particularly during their first conception, not only must avoid exercise in the first tri term, but should also take some natural herbs to protect their internal peace.

Q: Which exercises in this book could be done by a pregnant woman, or are you just referring to doing gentle movement in general?

Master Ni: After 7 to 8 months, some simple *Chi Kung (Chi Gong)* movement is all right, if you only do the amount you feel is safe and do not upset the womb. I think that if you do *Chi Kung (Chi Gong)*, a natural, easy delivery can be expected, because you have become physically fit. However, I do not think it is suitable to ride a motorcycle on a mountain ridge or in a wild field. A pregnant woman should walk to help keep herself healthy and strong.

---

[4]Master Ni has already given details of women's cultivation in many books, especially *Mystical Universal Mother* and *Mysticism*.

Q: Should a woman who is not physically strong start learning exercise by doing Chi Kung (Chi Gong)?

Master Ni: Yes, that is good.

Q: Is there any change that a woman needs to make during the time of menopause?

Master Ni: That is a great time for a woman. After menopause, a woman becomes almost neutral again, like a child before puberty. That is the benefit of menopause.

For purposes of spiritual cultivation, any gentle movement can be done, however gentle movement can also make the difficulty of menopause be over sooner. On the other hand, those practices can lengthen the youthfulness of the woman's body if done correctly and regularly. This is also true for men.

I particularly recommend that my women friends read the book about my mother.[5] If they are inspired by the women teachers who lived before or after my mother, I think they will be able to develop much more detailed knowledge than I can.

Q: Is Gentle Path T'ai Chi *Movement suitable for women?*

Master Ni: Gentle Path *T'ai Chi* works with the center of gravity below the waist. It gives a solid foundation that can take you in any direction you may wish to go: martial arts, physical health or spiritual development.

A woman's center is already low. Women can practice Gentle Path, but they should not squat or bend too low. I recommend that women focus on the Middle *Tan Tien* as their foundation. Because Sky Journey is in the middle range of speed and height, it is suitable. This exercise is adaptable to all kinds of people. Men and women of all ages can safely cultivate the Middle *Tan Tien*.

People with Special Health Considerations

Master Ni: Many people pant, become dizzy and sweat when they walk upstairs. Those are all symptoms of lack of correct exercise.

---

[5]*Mystical Universal Mother.*

Gentle movement can correct all such problems and improve your stamina. You will also enjoy yourself.

Q: If a person's health is not good, can they still learn? Is it inadvisable for someone in poor physical condition to exercise?

Master Ni: First they need to work on psychologically, emotionally and spiritually removing the negative conditions they have established throughout their lives. Such conditions are constant self-suggestions to become old and weak, so you cannot expect immediate results. They need to restore pure, fresh-mindedness first. This is why I recommend that all my young friends read my books. They are not the product of my individual effort but represent the achievement of all ancient achieved ones. Although they did not put their energy into writing books, at least we share the same energy of immortality.

Q: What exercise should be selected if someone has special health considerations?

Master Ni: People with high blood pressure should not do anything vigorous that would pump blood up into the head area. Someone who is overweight should take a lot of walks instead of sitting still all day. In general, I think people with health considerations need correct herbal or acupuncture treatment to improve their physical foundation. The mind and the body both need to be improved before pursuing any spiritual ambition, including the grace of God's salvation.

Q: Are you saying that a person has to already be in good physical and mental condition before starting to learn any of these exercises?

Master Ni: People need to adjust, depending on their degree of health. Some therapeutic *Chi Kung* (*Chi Gong*) is a medicine in itself. Some of you also might be interested in the audio cassette, *Chi Gong* for Pain Management.

By the way, if you are not used to exercising, do not try to do too much at once. Do what is not too difficult for you, and build yourself up slowly through consistent practice.

If you experience pain when practicing any of the movements, stop doing that movement. A little discomfort is all right, but pain is a warning. If you have any question about whether a particular exercise or movement is all right for you, consult your physician.

Q: Should you practice chi *movement such as* T'ai Chi *if you have a cold or the flu?*

Master Ni: No, you should totally relax. Do not do *Chi Kung (Chi Gong)* or meditation or *T'ai Chi*. A cold is a sign for you to rest. It is not necessarily an illness, but it is good to drink some warm herb tea.

People Interested in Martial Arts Training

Master Ni: If you consider *T'ai Chi* movement as a martial art, you must realize that there are secrets to learning both. The martial arts of the internal school are not for fighting, but for refining energy to attain *chi*. *Chi* or energy has different levels, but *chi* is everything in the universe. As a small model of nature, *chi* is our individual life. It changes, but it lasts.

As I have said before, practitioners of martial arts typically do not live long, even if they have achieved excellence in their art. They were trained with quickness, slowness, hardness and softness, which puts them in control when they enter combat. They take advantage of their training to become a champion. Expecting to be a martial arts champion and also have a long and happy life is like trying to have your cake and eat it too.

Q: Do martial arts help a person's health in any way?

Master Ni: Martial arts can be done for health and for fun, or for self-confidence. It does not have to make you into a warrior in the negative sense. The most highly achieved practitioners of martial arts are actually non-aggressive, yielding and tolerant. That is the true value of deep physical training in the ancient martial arts.

Q: Do you have advice for anyone wishing to learn martial arts?

Master Ni: Some types of martial arts do not build health, they only produce hot tempers. I suggest that everyone who practices martial arts also do some internal art to balance themselves and broaden their scope of using the body. No one can always sing high notes. Bruce Lee, the Chinese martial arts star, was an example of this. Consider your true goals. Do you want to control others or discipline yourself? Do you want to fight others or live in harmony with them?

Q: Some say that martial arts develop self-confidence and discipline.

Master Ni: I agree with that. I heard about a church that teaches youngsters how to shoot in order to build their confidence. I do not think that is the best or most effective way. Martial arts is good for young people who are too emotional or who have overly strong imaginations. For them, martial arts can be a great help.

Q: There are many styles of martial arts, such as Tae Kwando, Aikido, Ju Jitsu, Karate, *etc. Is one style better than another?*

Master Ni: Basically, they are the same tea by different names. Practices such as *Tae Kwando, Aikido, Ju Jitsu,* and *Karate* are taught to groups as an educational system. Social promotion does not express the essence.

For something as deep as the schools of *Wu Tang* or *Shao Lin* Temple, you need to find a good teacher, because such arts are a personal achievement. Achieved ones usually hid from the public and never told anyone what they had learned. Not because it was so secret, they just did not like to show off. As the proverb says: the half bottle of vinegar makes the most noise. It is important to learn from a teacher in order to achieve depth.

Good teachers are moderate. They never tell you how highly achieved they are. When you study with an achieved teacher, you are not just learning the form, you are learning the spirit of the teacher. The real value of whatever you learn depends on how good the teacher is. Some teachers are too business oriented, and their spiritual achievement is thin. They are more concerned with their own personal style than with the subtle universal truth.

Q: Is it good to learn martial arts for self-defense?

Master Ni: You cannot learn self-defense from martial arts alone. The best self-defense is the spiritual philosophy of being like a hen rather than a rooster. If you study martial arts for a long time, it may cause you to become too confident and think you are the strongest man in the world. This can cause you to push yourself to the verge of peril.

I only recommend martial arts as a spiritual cultivation, whether *Shao Lin* (the hard) or *Wu Tang* (the soft). This is the general way Chinese people distinguish them, as hard or soft. The *Shao Lin* School originally taught martial arts for spiritual purposes, but unfortunately it has become degraded into a tradition of combat. *Wu Tang*, which developed in the Wu Tang mountains was Master Tsan, San Fong's tradition. He got the idea from Master Chen Tuan's concept of *T'ai Chi*. Thus, *Wu Tang* has a more clear spiritual tradition, which I prefer.

Busy People With Little Time for Learning and Exercise

Q: Do you have any recommendations for people who are too busy to take a class?

Master Ni: Many students who work at home or in the office watch videos and do it in between intervals of work.

Q: Is any one of these exercises easier or faster to learn and thus more suitable for very busy people?

Master Ni: *Dao-In* and Eight Treasures are the easiest. Some people might also be interested in the audio cassette, *Chi Gong* for Stress Management.

Other Special Circumstances

Master Ni: If you are looking for expansion in your life and learning, learn *Dao-In*, Eight Treasures, Harmony/Trinity *T'ai Chi*, Gentle Path *T'ai Chi*, Sky Journey *T'ai Chi*, Infinite Expansion *T'ai Chi* and Cosmic Tour *Ba Gua Zahn*. If you keep doing them over the years, not only will you expand, but you will also forget how old you are.

If you wish to retreat from the world, first give up all external physical training and only practice gentle physical arts. Reduce the hours you do Infinite Expansion, then Sky Journey, Cosmic Tour, Gentle Path, Harmony/Trinity, and the Eight Treasures.

Increase the hours you do meditation, but do not become like a block of wood or stone. Do not cease practicing basic physical arts such as *Dao-In* and other gentle practices. These physical arts have levels of depth. When you reach that depth, it becomes part of your meditation. The benefit of different movements and practices will naturally become self-evident.

Dr. Daoshing Ni: One might ask, "Can one learn the physical arts without a teacher?" If one takes his or her learning seriously, and carefully follows the instructions in this book, the self-learning process will be quite successful. To have a teacher nearby, of course, has advantages over being self-taught, but it does not mean that self-learning is not possible. As a matter of fact, many famous teachers are self-taught. As long as one is diligent and follows the rules, continuous practice and learning will benefit both mental and physical health. A teacher can correct one's movements and assist one in learning more accurately and faster.

Q: I have been told that a good form of T'ai Chi *itself can be your teacher.*

Master Ni: That is right. I have learned many things, but most of them are passing attractions. The things I teach in this book have been refined through generations and they have taught me a lot through the years.

In most people's lives, the mind is dominant. If you have a good mind, you can recognize that the body can sometimes be your teacher. From its teaching or warning, you can apply your-self to another aspect of life and benefit from it. Thus, the teacher is not far.

Being an acupuncturist is a different energy or habit that can support and enable you to become a good healer. People who practice boxing, weight lifting, gymnastics and sports produce energy, but it is not healing energy. Healing energy is much deeper than muscular energy. Almost all medical professions, not only acupuncturists but also surgeons, dentists, etc., require dexterity. Sports affect how you manage yourself and can make you unable to fulfill certain skills gracefully or suitably. This is why learning *T'ai Chi* or *Chi Kung* (*Chi Gong*) is recommended for all types of healing professions. For people with spiritual interest and a delicate profession, practicing any of these arts is a cultivation that will assist your development and probably bring about the breakthrough you have been working on for many years.

Summary

Master Ni: Although different teachers have different emphases, all *T'ai Chi* forms follow the same basic principle. Choose any form that fits your natural inclinations, and you will increase your health and fitness. Increased health and fitness are the foundation of success.

All *T'ai Chi* forms have value, so you should not develop strong preferences or prejudices about them. Perfecting a particular style is a matter of artistic standard, not a universal standard of truth.

In the next chapter, I will discuss the different forms in further detail.

Chapter 3

Description of Each Type of Exercise

Dao-In (and Meditation)

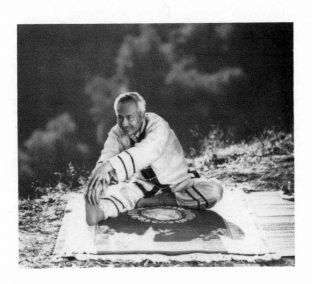

Dao-In
Purpose: Happiness, longevity and self-attunement
Center: The whole body
Goal: No physical trouble

Master Ni: *Dao-In* (pronounced dow-een) is a series of movements that have traditionally been called "exercises for conducting physical energy." It is a collection of exercises, somewhat similar to *hatha yoga*, from achieved masters who practiced indoors on a mat. Wise people tried to find a practical way to improve the stagnation of physical energy. For example, if you lie down too long, when you get up you will be stiff, or part of your body will be sore. If you walk, stand, sit or do physical work for too long, certain muscles, or the muscles of the entire body, will react. This includes tendons, cartilage and bones. The principle of *Dao-In* is to make adjustments to your body as necessary. When you get up and do a few movements, the internal flow of energy is affected and stagnation can be prevented.

Once people began doing this physical energy conducting, they discovered that it not only prevented stagnation, but it also improved their health and lengthened their life. Externally, it helps the muscles, tendons and bones. Internally, it helps different systems of the body function better, including the circulation, secretions and so forth. Its pure purpose is to nurture and attune your internal energy.

When you do *Dao-In*, the most important thing is relaxation. Some postures require more training of some of your muscles, so follow the principle of building your practice up slowly.

While it adjusts and attunes, *Dao-In* also generates, strengthens and invigorates your energy. There are five major parts to the whole system, three of which are the physical foundation. Another part is a meditation, and the concluding part is primarily focused on the face and head.

It takes about 30 minutes to perform the entire sequence of movements, but it is not necessary to do the entire set.

FOR A SELECTION OF *DAO-IN* EXERCISES, PLEASE SEE CHAPTER 15. FOR MORE INFORMATION, PLEASE SEE MASTER NI'S BOOK *ATTUNE YOUR BODY WITH DAO-IN* AND ITS COMPANION VIDEOTAPE.

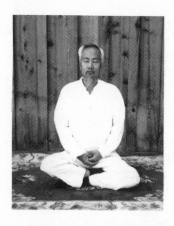

<u>Meditation</u>
Purpose: Uniting the mind with the body
Center: Middle *Tan Tien*
Goal: Gathering energy

Master Ni: Meditation is one aspect of self-cultivation and an important part of spiritual self-improvement. Meditation is sometimes a harvest, and at other times a refinement.

When practicing meditation, there must be no skepticism about what you are doing. If you are skeptical, you cannot meditate in quietude with pure energy. Being centered and all-embracing is the basic spiritual practice called *wu wei,* which is described in the *Tao Teh Ching.* Doing nothing extra may be the most fundamental of all virtues, and the highest. This is a simple reference to meditation as a form of sitting, walking or standing *Chi Kung (Chi Gong).*

FOR MORE DETAILED INFORMATION ON THE PRACTICE OF MEDITATION, PLEASE SEE *WORKBOOK FOR SPIRITUAL DEVELOPMENT OF ALL PEOPLE, ATTUNE YOUR BODY WITH DAO-IN* AND *SPRING THUNDER: AWAKEN THE HIBERNATING POWER OF YOUR LIFE.*

Eight Treasures

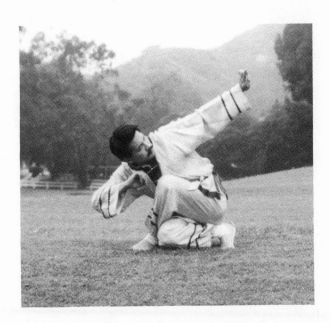

Purpose: Stimulating and accelerating the body's energy
Center: Upper, Middle and Lower *Tan Tien*
Goal: Strengthening the bodily kingdom

Master Ni: A beginning student of oriental styles of exercise might be interested in learning the Eight Treasures. It provides a good foundation for health, coordination and spirit.

In my heritage, the Eight Treasures are called *"Pa Kun Dao In"* 入公導引 which means "Channeling Exercise of the Eight Old Respectable Ones" or *"Shien Jia Ba Jin Tu"* 仙家八景圖, which means "Eight Groups of Exercise from the Immortal School." It has been nicknamed *"Ba Duan Jin,"* 八段錦.

The Eight Treasures are a form of *Dao-In* that was passed down from the Yellow Emperor through 74 generations of direct lineage in the tradition of the Integral Way to myself. They are a series of short exercises patterned after natural movements which, unlike *Dao-In*, are done standing up. Names such as "White Crane Washes Its Feathers" and "Move the Stars and Turn the Big Dipper" suggest a type of internal exercise (*Chi Kung* or *Chi Gong).*

You do not have to be in excellent athletic condition to do Eight Treasures. They are not as complicated as *T'ai Chi* Movement, but it is not necessary to do complicated arts. Complication is only an expression of athletic condition or talent.

Dr. Maoshing Ni: The Eight Treasures can be practiced by anyone at any level of fitness. People with severe health problems can benefit from practicing the method of breathing and placing less emphasis on the physical aspect. As one's health improves, the more physical part of the exercises can be emphasized. Those who are already in excellent physical condition can benefit by developing a strong center (abdominal *chi*) and a more harmonious flow of energy.

Certain *Chi Kung* (*Chi Gong)* styles emphasize different aspects or parts of the body. The Eight Treasures work not only on all parts of the body, but they activate all twelve channels and the eight extraordinary channels. Other *Chi Kung* (*Chi Gong)* styles may be limited to activating only certain channels.

It takes between 20 and 50 minutes to perform the entire sequence of movements, depending on how many repetitions you do and your speed. For several sample Eight Treasures movements, see Chapter 15. For more information and step-by-step instruction, please see Dr. Maoshing Ni's videotape and its companion book, *The Eight Treasures: Energy Enhancement Exercise.*

Crane Style *Chi Gong*

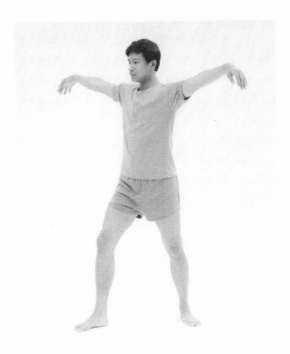

Purpose: Health
Center: According to instruction
Goal: Improve health and the nervous system

Dr. Daoshing Ni: Crane Style *Chi Gong* was developed by Dr. Zhao Jin Xian in September, 1980, in Beijing. Since then its popularity has spread throughout China. Every day, more and more people are practicing it to cure chronic ailments or simply for the joy of staying healthy.

In the Orient, especially in China, Korea and Japan, the crane symbolizes longevity and peacefulness. It has a quiet, non-competitive character. The movements of Crane Style *Chi Gong* are based on those of the crane, which are graceful and harmonious like the water of a mountain stream. Crane Style *Chi Gong* is simple to learn and practice. As long as one's mind follows the flow of *chi* during the exercise, its therapeutic effect is pronounced and one's energy becomes better regulated and balanced.

Each section of Crane Style *Chi Gong* concentrates on moving *chi* to a different area, opening up different points and strengthening the *chi* flow throughout various meridians. A brief summary of each of the six sections will help explain the energetic movements.

Section 1: The main purpose is to allow the body's internal *chi* to communicate with the environment or to take in fresh energy from the universe and expel stale energy from the body.
Section 2: The purpose is to open up the three *yang* meridians and three *yin* meridians on the hands.
Section 3: This set is used to regulate the flow of *chi* in the *Ren* and *Du* channels by loosening the vertebrae, thus causing the *yang chi* to rise and the *yin chi* to sink.
Section 4: This series is practiced to release stagnation in the upper and lower limbs and improve *chi* circulation.
Section 5: The main purpose of this standing meditation and ending section is to regulate the mind, the respiration, and the body (or, in other words, concentration, breathing, and posture).

Crane-Style *Chi Gong* is a balanced, nourishing practice which not only strengthens and refines your *chi*, but can also bring about a marked improvement in almost every aspect of your life.

CRANE STYLE *CHI GONG* IS A STANDING EXERCISE. ITS SLOW AND GRACEFUL MOVEMENTS DO NOT REQUIRE GREAT PHYSICAL EFFORT. IT TAKES ABOUT 20 MINUTES TO PERFORM THE ENTIRE SEQUENCE.

FOR A REPRESENTATIVE MOVEMENT OF CRANE STYLE *CHI GONG*, SEE CHAPTER 15. FOR MORE INFORMATION, PLEASE SEE DR. DAOSHING NI'S BOOK *CRANE STYLE CHI GONG* AND ITS COMPANION VIDEOTAPE.

Self-Healing *Chi Gong*

Purpose: Therapeutic
Center: According to the problem
Goal: General health

Dr. Maoshing Ni: Many *Chi Kung (Chi Gong)* exercises are designed for general health improvement and maintenance, but

Self-Healing *Chi Gong* is specifically therapeutic. Self-Healing *Chi Gong* consists of basic, simple exercises for each organ system of the body, and its effects are immediate.

The advantage of this system is that it gives people tools that empower them to help themselves. It is a self-regulating technique, similar to self-administered acupressure for a headache, the flu or a cough. All disease begins with a small imbalance. Self-Healing *Chi Gong* helps you become more in tune with and accountable for your own health.

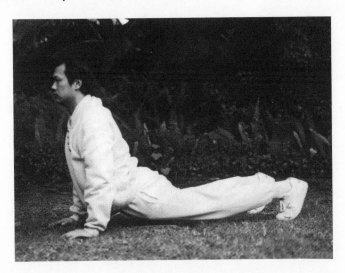

The five movements are: stomach strengthening, liver cleansing, kidney fortifying, lung/immunity boosting and heart circulating. For example, if someone gets into a heated argument and becomes so upset that he or she cannot calm down, cannot eat, has a headache, and is very nervous, that person can practice the liver cleansing movement, which will drain the anger away within minutes.

Another example is someone who experiences bloating, distension and gas pains after eating. Instead of popping pills, the person can practice the stomach strengthening movement and experience relief in a short time. Self-Healing *Chi Gong* is easy to learn and use.

FOR INSTRUCTIONS ON HOW TO DO *SELF-HEALING CHI GONG*, PLEASE SEE
DR. MAOSHING NI'S VIDEOTAPE BY THAT NAME. YOU MIGHT ALSO BE INTER-
ESTED IN THE AUDIO CASSETTES, *CHI GONG FOR STRESS RELEASE* AND *CHI GONG
FOR PAIN MANAGEMENT*.

Harmony/Trinity *T'ai Chi* Movement

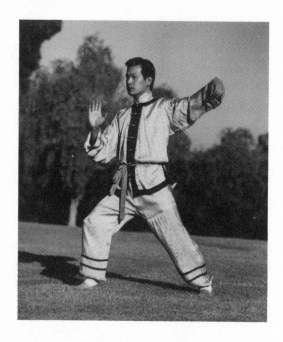

Purpose: Coordination of the entire body
Center: All three *Tan Tien*
Goal: Balancing the energy

Master Ni: There are many styles of *T'ai Chi* being taught in Taiwan
and China today. Harmony/Trinity is similar to those styles, yet it
maintains a gracefulness, naturalness and evenness that exceeds
any of the newer styles. As its name implies, it brings about unity
between the body, mind and spirit. It is a good practice for people
of any age for health, enjoyment and artistic intention. It is the
most suitable style for people who admire and would like to learn
some simple *T'ai Chi*.

In my teaching of the Integral Way, the path of spiritual self-development, the Eight Treasures is required, along with Harmony/Trinity *T'ai Chi*. Other styles of *T'ai Chi* are not required, because they are for more advanced students who have a higher interest, ambition or enjoyment.

Harmony/Trinity *T'ai Chi* Movement (also called Unity Movement) contains the essence of the *Chen, Yang* and *Wu* styles. *Chen* movement was developed earlier than *Yang* and *Wu*, which are later, simplified styles. The *Chen* Style, which alternates between strength and softness, originally developed from martial arts. The *Yang* Style tends to be gentle and slow. The *Wu* Style tends to be lighter and faster.

Harmony/Trinity *T'ai Chi* movement is not a particularly popular style, because it does not emphasize the Lower *Tan Tien*, although it definitely strengthens the Lower *Tan Tien*. It is suitable for men or women of all ages, and Dr. Maoshing Ni has produced a videotape of it.

Dr. Maoshing Ni: Trinity Style *T'ai Chi* captures the gracefulness and the meditative benefits of the popular *Yang* Style, the power generating aspects of the *Chen* Style, and the agility of the *Wu* Style. It distills the unique benefits of all three styles into one form that can be easily learned by anyone who is interested in improving their health and well-being. Many serious students may learn Trinity Style as a stepping stone to the higher forms of *T'ai Chi* Movement such as Gentle Path, Sky Journey or Infinite Expansion.

HARMONY/TRINITY *T'AI CHI* IS A STANDING MOVEMENT, DONE FASTER THAN CRANE STYLE *CHI GONG* WITH MOVEMENTS THAT ARE MORE SEQUENTIAL THAN THE EIGHT TREASURES. IT TAKES ABOUT 40 MINUTES TO PERFORM THE ENTIRE FORM.

FOR MORE INFORMATION, PLEASE SEE DR. MAOSHING NI'S VIDEOTAPES *T'AI CHI CHUAN I AND II*.

Gentle Path *T'ai Chi* Movement

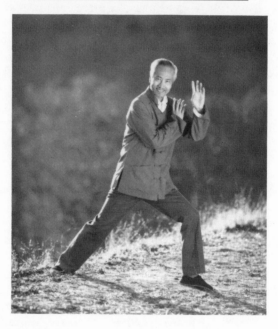

Purpose: Strengthen and refine the hormonal system
Center: Lower *Tan Tien*
Goal: Control and refinement of sexual desire[6]

Master Ni: Gentle Path *T'ai Chi* movement focuses on nurturing the Lower *Tan Tien*, which is the central point between the navel and the sexual organs. This area is connected with the breath. Have you ever observed how you and other people breathe? When a baby breathes, the whole cavity of the baby's trunk, from its shoulders down to its legs, stretches and contracts. The Lower *Tan Tien* works together with the lungs to allow the baby to breathe fully. However, as most people grow older, their breath becomes shorter and shorter until it can barely fill the lungs any more. That is dangerous, because the Lower *Tan Tien* is the center of natural vitality in most people. This is especially true of men and physical workers. Although today more people do intellectual work, their

---

[6]For further information, see *Workbook for Spiritual Development,* "Invocation for Dual Cultivation."

vitality still relies on the Lower *Tan Tien*.

Each movement of Gentle Path *T'ai Chi* tonifies the Lower *Tan Tien*, which in turn strengthens and enlivens you. Deep, full breathing while doing the exercise is another fortifying factor. All areas in the abdominal cavity produce vital energy that stays in the organs.

Sometimes the pattern of these movements is stretching and gathering. When you stretch, your energy moves throughout your whole body. When you contract or gather, the energy returns to the center of your body. It requires time and practice, good control and awareness of your breathing to become effective and precise in coordinating your energy with the movements.

Why is this exercise called Gentle Path? Because it is based on the principles of the *Tao Teh Ching*, which teaches us how to be gentle in our lives. It also teaches us to be nonviolent in our emotions, in our personal attitudes and in our physical actions. Many people understand the value of being gentle, but they cannot be that way unless they have achieved internal harmony.

General education uses intellectual knowledge as a tool. People know and tell each other to be gentle, but it is more important to be able to do it in your life. The physical and spiritual education you receive from doing this gentle exercise will help you stay calm in rough situations and handle them gently and smoothly. That is only one of its many benefits.

GENTLE PATH *T'AI CHI* IS SOMETIMES CALLED THE EARTH STYLE OR STYLE OF WISDOM.

GENTLE PATH IS A STANDING MOVEMENT, DONE FASTER THAN CRANE STYLE *CHI GONG* WITH MOVEMENTS THAT ARE MORE SEQUENTIAL THAN THE EIGHT TREASURES. IT TAKES ABOUT 40 MINUTES TO PERFORM THE ENTIRE SEQUENCE.

TO OBSERVE GENTLE PATH *T'AI CHI* MOVEMENT AND THE OTHER TWO TYPES OF *T'AI CHI* MOVEMENT, PLEASE SEE MASTER NI'S VIDEOTAPE, *T'AI CHI CHUAN: AN APPRECIATION*. FOR COMPLETE INSTRUCTIONS FOR LEARNING GENTLE PATH, PLEASE SEE MASTER NI'S VIDEOTAPE, *GENTLE PATH T'AI CHI CHUAN*, EXPECTED TO BE AVAILABLE AFTER SUMMER OF 1996.

Sky Journey *T'ai Chi* Movement

Purpose: Uniting with nature
Center: Middle *Tan Tien*
Goal: Soften the body and increase the *chi*

Master Ni: Sky Journey's central focus is the Middle *Tan Tien*, which is located in the thoracic cavity at the point between the nipples (the heart area). The Middle *Tan Tien* is one of the places where you gather energy. Because this exercise was specifically designed and structured to be high, with the center in the Middle *Tan Tien*, it is not suitable to squat or bend too low while doing it. It should be done with the body gently erect and with the knees straight or only slightly bent.

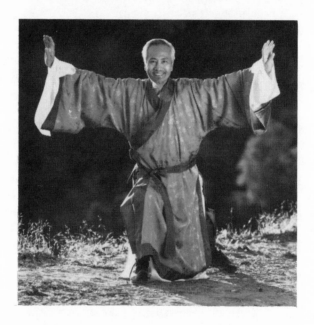

According to natural cosmology, human beings are the middle point in universal development between the physical world and the spiritual world. Without human life, the energies of Heaven and Earth would be separate and have no chance to meet each other. Your life is the bridge between Heaven and Earth.

Most of the movements of this exercise are for the purpose of energy conducting, although they once had a martial purpose. Their purpose now, however, is to defeat certain untamed parts of oneself. Sky Journey is a little faster than other *T'ai Chi* movements such as Gentle Path. It is in the middle range of speed, but it is still not the fastest. If you do it too fast, you will not perform the details correctly, and its effect will be lessened.

Sky Journey is suitable for all people, but it is especially suitable for women, because women generally benefit from maintaining their energy in the Middle *Tan Tien*. This exercise is also good for men of all ages, because the Middle *Tan Tien* is a safe spot to pay attention to and cultivate.

All practices have different purposes and goals. Sky Journey, as the middle way, can be a preparation for a further, higher learning. For example, you can use Sky Journey to pacify your emotions, or you can use it to excite and stimulate your body. You can also use it to go in the direction of learning the art of weapons or just do it for self-adjustment and self-control. From a central point, you can go anywhere.

The purpose of practicing the Sky Journey is to learn how to make smooth transitions in life. That is its main benefit, in addition to physical health. Doing this exercise, you can come closer to the Way than by only reading books.

SKY JOURNEY *T'AI CHI* IS ALSO REFERRED TO AS MANKIND STYLE OR STYLE OF HARMONY. IT TAKES APPROXIMATELY 20 MINUTES TO COMPLETE SKY JOURNEY *T'AI CHI* MOVEMENT.

TO OBSERVE SKY JOURNEY *T'AI CHI* MOVEMENT AND THE OTHER TWO TYPES OF *T'AI CHI* MOVEMENT, PLEASE SEE MASTER NI'S VIDEOTAPE, *T'AI CHI CHUAN: AN APPRECIATION*. FOR COMPLETE INSTRUCTIONS FOR LEARNING SKY JOURNEY, PLEASE SEE MASTER NI'S VIDEOTAPE, *SKY JOURNEY T'AI CHI CHUAN*, EXPECTED TO BE AVAILABLE AFTER AUTUMN OF 1996.

Infinite Expansion *T'ai Chi* Movement

Purpose: Self-generation of the body
Center: Upper *Tan Tien* and central axis
Goal: Self-authority over physical life and spontaneous response to danger

Master Ni: Infinite Expansion was previously called "The Heavenly Ladder," "Uniting with Heaven" or "The Style of Integration," all of which describe the motion of this exercise. When you practice it, you feel as though you are climbing clouds, because frequently you bend and bring your knee close to your abdomen like climbing a ladder. It also feels as though you are a bird in flight.

Infinite Expansion is very different from Gentle Path and Sky Journey. It is closer to martial art and can be excellent training in that regard. Infinite Expansion is thus practiced at a higher range and speed. It focuses on the axis that runs from the top of the head down the middle of the body to the perineum. The top of the head is called "Hundred Meeting" (*Du* 20 or *Baihui*), which is the meeting point of *yang* energy. The trunk of the human body basically has a rounded shape. The center of the body has an axis similar to that of the hub of a wheel, and the spokes all meet at the hub.

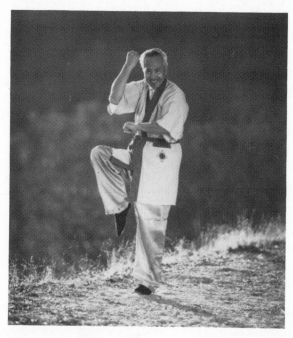

Infinite Expansion is considered the earliest form of *T'ai Chi* movement and is believed to have been taught by initiated masters and refined through generations before being passed down to us. It was a secret, high achievement in martial arts, taught only to a special few, not to aggressive students. In China, few people have the chance to learn it or understand it. I offer it to all people as an excellent form of physical training. High achievement depends on an individual's devotion.

You can practice Infinite Expansion while listening to good music as a background to help you move and lend a sense of recreation to the exercise. You feel great when you do it, as though you are reaching somewhere. Nothing else gives you the same experience with equal benefit. It can prevent you from aging fast, or even make you forget your age altogether. It is light and a delight. If your goal is to go beyond all limitations, you can achieve it through this exercise. However, you need to practice until you perfect it. First develop skill, then go beyond the skill to reach the heights of spiritual bliss.

In spiritual learning, we talk about unlimitedness or the infinite, but in practical worldly life we need limits. For example, you cannot talk without limits. If you do, people will not trust you any more. You cannot eat without limits. If you do, you will become obese. You cannot drink without limits. In China, the elders of almost every family drink rice wine in the wintertime. Rice wine is not like Japanese *sake*. *Sake* is thin and Chinese rice wine is thick. Thick wine is more tonifying and does not cause headaches. Older people usually consider rice wine a tonic, and they do not drink too much. However, if they go past healthy limits and drink unlimitedly, they become drunk.

So, whatever you do, it seems you must have limits. When I say, "you need to have limits," I mean you cannot go beyond what is healthy, useful, truthful, necessary or appropriate. If you do, you will make trouble for yourself. Having limits does not mean that people manage you. You learn to manage and control yourself. When you learn self-control, all your movements are proper and skillful in any situation.

Once you are achieved in Infinite Expansion, you are not limited by your physical body, and you can go beyond this set of movements. Some masters practice it devotedly. It was recorded that one master, in his old age, could do this art in the snow without leaving a trace. That is going beyond physical law. Some masters achieved invisibility. This is also a spiritual practice.

There are three aspects to Infinite Expansion movement. The first is self-control, the second is the whirlpool formation of the energy, and the third is internal energy surfing. An untrained eye might not be able to see those subtleties, so I am explaining them to you. I hope that once you understand these points, you will be inspired to practice.

Infinite Expansion has another interesting aspect, which is the tradition of spiritual swordsmanship. That tradition has an invocation that is used as a spiritual practice. I was told that if you practice that invocation, you will receive energy from nature. Generally, the art of movement is enough and complete in itself.

The practice of Infinite Expansion is suitable for anyone who has learned other *T'ai Chi* movements. The specific value of Infinite Expansion is its circular or cyclical movements. All movements that appear to move outward actually follow a spiral of going out and then retreating.

I have practiced Infinite Expansion more than the other styles, because it is so convenient. It can be done in a big or a small space. A space as small as the top of a dining table is big enough.

In ancient times, it was not allowed to show Infinite Expansion movement to others. Anyone who saw it might think it was a martial art and would challenge the peace-seeking practitioner to a fight, so he usually stayed indoors to avoid trouble. Of course, if you practice indoors, you should open a window to let in fresh air. In modern times, it is okay to do it outdoors, because now people will usually not challenge you.

The flow of energy in Infinite Expansion is like the ocean; you can go everywhere, endlessly. You go beyond, and nothing can restrain you. Have you experienced infinity? Infinity can be experienced in movement or in quietude. What does infinity mean? Dear friends, you must find out for yourselves. To do so is a challenge and a training. From your practice, you may reach infinity.

IT TAKES ABOUT 20 MINUTES TO PERFORM INFINITE EXPANSION ON BOTH THE LEFT AND RIGHT SIDES.

TO OBSERVE INFINITE EXPANSION *T'AI CHI* MOVEMENT AND THE OTHER TWO STYLES OF *T'AI CHI* MOVEMENT, PLEASE SEE MASTER NI'S VIDEOTAPE, *T'AI CHI CHUAN: AN APPRECIATION*. FOR COMPLETE INSTRUCTIONS FOR LEARNING INFINITE EXPANSION, PLEASE SEE MASTER NI'S VIDEOTAPE, *INFINITE EXPANSION T'AI CHI CHUAN*, EXPECTED TO BE AVAILABLE AFTER WINTER OF 1996.

Walking

Purpose: Gentle stimulation, with the soles touching the ground
Center: Nature
Goal: Health enhancement

Master Ni: It is good to take a walk before and after you do *T'ai Chi*. Do not be superstitious and consider *T'ai Chi* the only exercise you can do. Do not forget to walk. I have seen many masters who enjoyed *T'ai Chi* and became champions in fighting, but they forgot about walking, so that is not properly doing *T'ai Chi*. They did not know how to let the energy burn properly, so they became fat and did not do well.

Unfortunately you cannot do *T'ai Chi* all the time in daily life, because it is inconvenient. If you do *T'ai Chi* on a busy street, you attract a crowd and cannot concentrate as well. Thus, to keep training, you must also walk. Because your legs and arms alternate in their movements, walking follows the principle of *t'ai chi,* which is the alternating movement of *yin* and *yang.*

T'ai Chi practice should only be done for about 20 minutes or slightly longer. If you overdo it, you become overly electrified, which means the *chi* is too strong. A suitable amount of electrical energy becomes healthy vitality. A well-trained practitioner of *T'ai Chi Chuan* can knock a person out ten yards away because the electrical current temporarily numbs the opponent's heart so that he loses control. So do not do too much *T'ai Chi*. If you take a walk, you can go much longer than just 20 minutes and also be very peaceful. Do not think that *T'ai Chi* can replace walking.

Surely there is more benefit from *T'ai Chi* than from general walking, but combining *T'ai Chi* practice with walking will bring better all around results.

WALKING CAN BE PRACTICED FOR ANY LENGTH OF TIME AND AT ANY SPEED. FOR HAND POSTURES WITH WALKING, PLEASE SEE THE DESCRIPTION OF MERRY-GO-ROUND.

Cosmic Tour *Ba Gua Zahn* and Merry-Go-Round

Cosmic Tour
Purpose: Extending the physical nature to spiritual nature
Center: Lower *Tan Tien* with energy reaching to all points
Goal: Enjoyment of the cosmology of natural movement: "I move, so the universe moves."

Merry-Go-Round (for photos, please see Chapter 15)
Purpose: Joy in practice
Center: All three *Tan Tien*
Goal: A happy relationship between the emotional and physical aspects

Master Ni: In recent years, some communities and hospitals in China organized a test to compare the results and effects of doing Cosmic Tour to other kinds of exercise and sports. The results showed that Cosmic Tour is outstanding for the purposes of healing, rehabilitation and preventive maintenance.

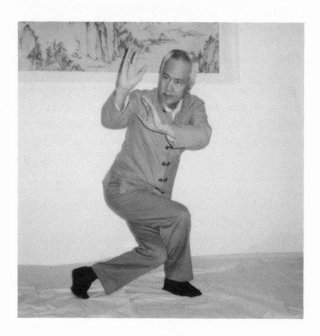

As a physical art, Cosmic Tour is not only movement, it is also a body language for spiritual communication with yourself. If you practice it, you will learn to unite and develop your whole body, not just your intellect or your physical strength. For example, a dancer who waves a streamer of colored silk in the air is one with her cloth. Similarly, in Cosmic Tour you move your whole body, not only on the physical level but also on the more subtle levels.

In Cosmic Tour, the circular movement resembles the spiritual maturity of an individual's personality. A mature person will not hit an obstruction but will go around it to avoid friction or damage. Circular movement is the cosmological framework of the universe and life. Because their orbits are defined, heavenly bodies do not collide and thus find endless life and infinite transformation.

The whole set of movements in Cosmic Tour is based on continuous rotation in many directions. Many circles, big and small, are made. This is why it is called Cosmic Tour. The sixty-four movements of Cosmic Tour were developed according to the principles expressed in the *Book of Changes* and its sixty-four hexagrams.

As you go around the circle of Cosmic Tour, you may feel happy, relaxed and graceful. When changing direction or changing from one posture to another, a kind of twisting motion occurs. One student fondly referred to this set of movements as "the twister," because the hands, arms, body, muscles and tendons all twist. Alternate twisting and relaxing gives the muscles a healthy workout. Most people do not know the benefits of such twisting movement, which is a natural body massage that goes much deeper than massaging muscle tissue.

Cosmic Tour is a special kind of exercise that developed from walking meditation.[7] You walk a while, then make a change by twisting your body. You relax during the walking. General *T'ai Chi* movement or other martial arts do not have such pauses for gentle walking, but this style of movement adjusts internal tension and relaxes the breath. Alternate exercise and repose is a different pattern of spiritual cultivation. This is why I include this set of exercises along with *T'ai Chi* and *Dao-In*.

Once a master said, "Do *T'ai Chi* for other people, but do Cosmic Tour for yourself." In saying that, she meant that *T'ai Chi* is a graceful movement that people enjoy watching, but Cosmic Tour is something to do for oneself, not to perform for people. Internal movement is not suitable for public performance. For example, *T'ai Chi* movement, which is similar to a martial art form, is an internal practice, but it is more performable than Cosmic Tour, which is almost completely internal. Cosmic Tour is more suitable for private practice or for a small group of dedicated people.

People who experience dizziness or suffer recurrent headaches due to congestion would benefit from doing more backward walking movement in this practice. This can also aid throbbing or pulsation of the heart. If you have a tendency towards high blood pressure or a stroke, regular slow practice will help.

---

[7]For a description of walking meditation, see *The Workbook for Spiritual Development of All People*, page 148 of the first edition or page 136 of the revised edition.

The original Cosmic Tour was simple, mostly just walking. You may go one step beyond simple walking and add the hand positions described as the Merry-Go-Round in the book *Power of Natural Healing* and in the exercise description in this book.

Cosmic Tour exemplifies the Eight Great Manifestations of nature that are expressed as different energies in the *Book of Changes*, which is also called the *I Ching*. The *Book of Changes* explains the eight arrangements of natural energy in great depth. The pleasure and benefit you receive from the philosophy of the *I Ching* with the Eight Great Manifestations can be expanded by doing the Cosmic Tour. Are we not making a cosmic tour in our lifetime when we physically enter the world?

It takes approximately 20 minutes to perform Merry-Go-Round, which is a simplified version of Cosmic Tour. It takes approximately 20 minutes to perform Cosmic Tour *Ba Gua Zahn*.

For more information about Cosmic Tour, please see Chapter 13.

For a simplified practice of Cosmic Tour *Ba Gua Zahn* which is called Merry-Go-Round, see Chapter 15 and also read *Power of Natural Healing*.

For complete instructions for learning Cosmic Tour, please see Master Ni's videotape, Cosmic Tour *Ba Gua Zahn*, expected to be available after the spring of 1997.

Martial Arts and Wu Shu

Includes Shao Lin *(the hard form, which is a formal martial art) and* Wu Tang *(the soft form, which may be only bodily adjustment), which are the two main schools, and* Karate, Tae Kwando, Ju Jitsu, Kung Fu, Judo *and* Aikido

Purpose: Fighting
Center: Muscular strength
Goal: To win

Besides being a physical art, *T'ai Chi* movement was often adapted to suit a special purpose. When a father and son needed to resist the invading Manchurians, and the inland farmers needed to protect themselves from the attack of maritime invaders, *T'ai Chi Chuan* was used as a martial art. Those special uses were necessary when violence and disorder prevailed.

Nevertheless, some teachers and practitioners are too serious about developing fighting skills. For the most part, martial arts movies that make fighting look glamorous are only choreographed dances. I do not think most martial arts can be applied in a real fight the way that a practitioner imagines they can. The greatest benefit of martial arts is self-confidence and health, not fighting skill. Dissolve your fantasies of glorious battles and just enjoy the movements. Practicing *T'ai Chi* with a martial arts intent detracts from the focus of the complete, pure teaching of the Way.

I

The Limitations of Martial Arts

Even if a person is good at push hands or has won championships, it is only when people play the same game by the same rules that you can be a better hand. In any game, including chess or martial arts, if you wish to win or do better than others, a certain set of rules must be observed. Only then can a person with good training and skill do better than others.

A young person may think very highly of his or her achievement in martial arts, but having such a skill is like sailing a small boat in a safe harbor. Later, you see that physical strength blocks you, because it has limitations. Only by using physical arts to learn the Way can one see the vastness and profundity of nonphysical natural power.

II

Winning and Losing

I learned that winning a battle, fight or game does not depend upon physical strength or specific achievement. It is the law of movement that determines whether or not you will win. The law of movement is not a human law; it is the utmost naturalness. The law of naturalness can only be known through practice and cultivation. With naturalness, in a situation of external pressure you will react without nervousness or exaggeration.

In simple words, the matter of winning is internal; so is the matter of losing. On a higher level, the real winner is not the person who fights in an arena, but the person who does not even watch the fight.

In the relative sphere of worldly life, there are winners and losers. One level of spiritual cultivation is to help oneself not be a total loser in life. Some people win because of superficial circumstances, but that is different from reaching the naturalness of their own life being. Superficial winning does not necessarily bring gain and superficial losing does not necessarily bring loss.

In reality, there are neither winners nor losers. The most important thing is to play well and keep moving forward without losing one's good spirits. The true winner is the one with a spirited life, no matter what the external circumstances.

It is hard to be oneself in competition, and difficult to ignore or refuse external influences in the general circumstances of life. Yet you can almost determine success or failure through your own achievement of the law of naturalness. You also have the freedom to walk away from a battle. It is easy to meet someone else's challenge by accepting a meaningless fight, but it is harder to walk away from it. That is high achievement. If you are relaxed about a situation because you understand it even if your opponent does not, then you have the power to walk away. The wise Yen Shi (the student of Lao Tzu) said, "If the blade of a knife is sharp, how can it harm you if you do not touch it?"

Some martial arts teachers are wise. They help you become so highly achieved in martial arts that you are no longer a fighting rooster. You become more interested in personal spiritual achievement than in fighting and winning. It is as though you were castrated, not in a negative sense but in the positive sense of having transformed the instinct for meaningless physical fights.

Being warlike is not just the tendency of a few individuals, it is a problem of human society. Spiritual development helps overcome this. To develop spiritually is to learn the Way.

III

Being Wise

The ancient sages changed the focus of gentle movement from martial arts toward a natural healthy life and intangible, infinite expansion. A wise person is not afraid to seem like a coward regarding the use of physical force. The wisdom of peacefulness takes skill, mental ability and grace.

If you desire it, a peaceful world awaits you, with no sort of fighting. The way to achieve it is to be peaceful yourself. That is why we practice the physical arts of the ancient achieved ones and study their helpful guidance to help us understand this truth more deeply.

Sword Practice

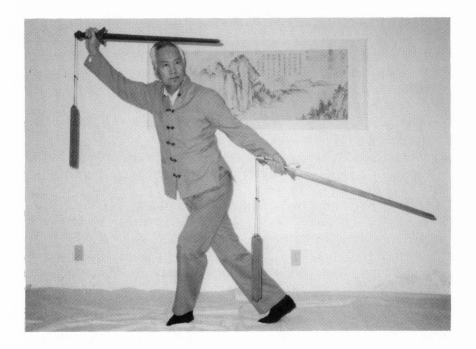

Purpose: Spiritual concentration
Center: Upper *Tan Tien*
Goal: Spiritual enhancement

Master Ni: At one stage of my life I liked all sword practice because it is much more graceful than general martial arts. I limit it to being my personal enjoyment as a form of spiritual cultivation on a level that transforms the spirit from my hormonal level to become *chi* and transfers the general physical *chi* to become *sen*, spiritual potency. With this in mind, I think that sword practice can be considered a spiritual practice.

As I view it, general sword dancing is for pleasure and has no spiritual meaning, although it has a lot of graceful postures and movements. It is great to watch women, children, or old people do a sword dance. If you use sword practice for spiritual purposes, however, then it will help your cultivation.

Chi Kung (*Chi Gong*), *Dao-In* and Eight Treasures can be the foundation on which practices such as Martial Arts, Sword Practice and Push Hands can be based.

In my school, the School of Internal Harmony, the sword is not used for fighting or fencing. It is for developing spiritual concentration. Having good spiritual concentration affects the health of your body, mind and spirit in a positive way.

FOR FURTHER INFORMATION ABOUT SPIRITUAL SWORDSMANSHIP, PLEASE SEE CHAPTER 14.

Push Hands

Purpose: An experience of the soft overcoming the strong
Center: Lower *Tan Tien*
Goal: Physical proof

Master Ni: Push hands is only one application of *T'ai Chi* movement. Under certain regulations, as one style of exercise or game, one can skillfully throw an opponent yards away. This can be one way of applying your achievement from practicing different *T'ai Chi* forms. Push hands is a game for young students and beginners, but it is not the final goal of *T'ai Chi* movement, which is to develop yourself integrally in all spheres.

In my 30s, I was a great fan of push hands, but my spiritual cultivation was a higher priority than anything else. Although push hands is an art, when you do it, you are naturally looking to win. You think about it, even in your sleep, until your muscles react to your imagination. I still have that bad habit. It has taken me many years to dissolve the concept of having an opponent, because when you do push hands you have an opponent. In contrast, when you learn the Way, you learn for absolute oneness, and thus you cannot have the concept of an opponent.

In one stage, push hands is useful for people who are too influenced by their own illusions. Why? If your mind is scattered, you will be defeated in push hands and knocked far away. Push hands is helpful in developing the power of concentration.

For more information about practicing martial arts, you might like to read my book *Tao, the Subtle Universal Law* because it has several relevant sections about the practice of *T'ai Chi*, especially Chapter 6.

Chapter Conclusion

You have an opportunity for success with *T'ai Chi* movement and *Chi Kung* (*Chi Gong*). One important element that can truly serve you is to have great confidence in what you have chosen to do by practicing it constantly. With practice and perseverance, you shall achieve your goals. Many people have attained a long and happy life, and I wish the same for you.

Whatever exercise or practice you choose to do, determination and regular practice will bring you far more emotional and spiritual benefit than only doing things like reading books, watching television and so forth.

The most essential teaching of the Integral Way is the knowledge of how to move internal power outwardly for a positive purpose. Practically, it is a training in fearlessness and healthy self-confidence. The most essential practice is to become "the one of universal self-responding truth within all people." Quite simply, it is the sound of "*Hon!*" (thunder). This means to ignore complications and just go ahead with your upright life!

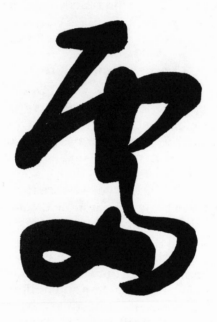

Hon!

Chapter 4

Guidelines for Practicing Movement

A young man traveled to a foreign land to attend the school of a famous teacher of Tao. When he arrived at the school he was interviewed by the teacher.

"What do you wish from me?" the teacher asked.

"I wish to be your student and become the finest Taoist in all the land," the man replied. "How long must I study?"

"A minimum of twenty years," the teacher answered.

"Twenty years is a long time," said the young man. "What if I studied twice as hard as all your other students?"

"Forty years," was the teacher's reply.

"Why is it that?" the puzzled young man asked.

"When one is fixated on the achievement, the mind becomes tight and one is further from the Way than before," responded the teacher.

Section 1: Introduction

Master Ni: In doing *T'ai Chi* movement and in living our lives, our goal is to be healthy and normal. Nothing special, just normal. The movement in *T'ai Chi* practice is a constant, healthy flow, not an erratic flow that is subnormal or abnormal.

Part of living a healthy, spiritual life includes being active in the morning and reposeful in the evening. A healthy schedule is good for your practice as well as for your health and overall well-being. Do those things that are of lasting benefit rather than short-lived advantage or immediate gratification.

A practitioner of self-cultivation practices endurance under pressure and maintains balance when there is no trouble. Therefore, an achieved one, like the center of the universe, is inexhaustible.

Our goal is to fully achieve ourselves while living within the inescapable network of worldly life. Other spiritual traditions claim that liberation means giving up worldly life to live as a hermit in the forests or as a beggar in the streets. That kind of liberation is only a futile attempt to escape from life. Life is an inescapable

network in which everyone is involved. True freedom from difficulties, be they conceptual, spiritual or physical, cannot be found
in an artificial lifestyle. A truly achieved person is someone whose
spirit is free, whatever the circumstances of life happen to be; in
other words, a healthy person who is able to rise above passing
troubles that have no real importance.

Doing *T'ai Chi* is so simple. When I describe it intellectually it
may sound complicated, but that is not the reality. When you truly
practice a gentle physical art such as *T'ai Chi* movement, it is not
just an exercise, it is life. In life, each moment and each action
expresses the same integral truth that *T'ai Chi* movement embodies
and expresses. Nothing can separate you or your actions from that
truth.

Section 2: General Instruction
Master Ni: To do physical arts successfully, certain internal
requirements must be observed and practiced, because the overall
purpose is internal. The internal and external elements of movement
are not really separate, although the movements of some forms of
T'ai Chi or *Chi Kung (Chi Gong)* can be learned one by one and
repeated over and over again before putting them together as a
whole form that creates a kind of atmosphere or situation.

Learning any art takes time and patience. Achieve it slowly. To
keep moving and exercising is what is important, because the
core of this art is your health.

A. Where to Practice
Master Ni: It is suitable to do this exercise in a park or your own
back or front yard, as long as there is no distraction from nearby
roads, thick dust, or people. Any quiet, undisturbed natural place
is suitable for internal energy cultivation. It is also all right to
practice indoors with the windows open for fresh air.

B. When to Practice
Master Ni: You might practice in the early morning before break-
fast. Most people go to work after that, but if you already have
material support and you have the chance, you might practice
again later in the day. The hours between 10:00 a.m. to 4:00 p.m.
and from 9:00 to 11:00 p.m. are when most people have a half-
empty stomach, so those are good times to do physical arts. If you

are an early bird and get up at 4:00 a.m., you can practice then. The later hours are for people with a different schedule.

Dr. Maoshing Ni: Spiritual practices are traditionally done in the early morning. In our modern, fast-paced society, however, *chi* exercise may be done at any time that is convenient for the individual.

Q: I do office work. I used to take a vigorous movement class in the evening, and only recently understood that exercising in the evening was causing problems. For example, it weakened my mind so that I had trouble doing things at work the next day; I even had trouble remembering what I was supposed to do. I would also have trouble waking up the morning after the class.
  On the other hand, if I exercise too much in the morning, I also have a hard time concentrating at work. I want to move around instead of sitting still.

Master Ni: For people who do mental work, the best time to exercise is from three to five o'clock in the afternoon, but not after five. Exercise about forty minutes before dinner, and then eat a light dinner. Do not overdo it in the morning either.
  Physical law and the law of mind are the same. For example, if you spend a lot of time thinking in the evening, it is hard to stop thinking when you sleep. Similarly, doing vigorous physical movement and then immediately sitting down is too rapid a change and can be damaging to the lungs and other organs because of the sudden internal pressure that has gathered.
  When you exercise in the morning, start very slowly and gently and then build up to a suitable speed later, but do not overly excite the body's energy, either in the morning or at night.
  I would like to comment on another point that is related to your question. Learning the forms by memorizing them is intellectual learning. We already have too much intellectual activity in modern life. A better way to learn is to follow the video and do it again and again. Over time, you will learn it naturally. It may take longer, but will be less burdensome mentally.
  When I was a child, I learned 4,000 types of herbs, over 1,000 acupuncture points, many kinds of diseases, and other specialized knowledge about Traditional Chinese Medicine. If you tried

to do that from memory, it might kill you. I learned it by using it. You learn it, you do it, you learn it, you do it, and by that method you pick it up gradually and unconsciously. The unconscious way of learning is much easier than conscious memorization. Too many people spoil their lives by overtaxing the conscious part of the mind.

Be natural. Being natural means learning or doing things without too much thought. Do not allow your mind to always take the lead. For example, if you have a particularly difficult problem, put it aside until the next day or some other time when you can respond to it in a natural way instead of punishing yourself by constantly thinking about it.

C. Posture and the Spine

Master Ni: I would like to share some special details on how to practice the physical arts. First, the spine should always be aligned, from the tailbone to where it joins the head, so that it is straight but not rigid like a drill instructor's posture. There should be a natural flexibility in its alignment. In some movements, the head is raised a little bit in order to adjust one's balance.

The internal school calls the spine "the dragon bone," or "the dragon," because it is the source of one's mental, physical and spiritual strength and also the means of communication between what is substantial and what is insubstantial. If the spine is not well aligned, the *chi* that flows through it moves poorly and one's health declines, because the powerful dragon is no longer active. A healthy spine is similar to the shape of a released or a slightly pulled bow.

There is a second detail to be remembered. The tailbone, including the sphincter muscle around the anus, should always be tucked forward. Also, the chin should also be kept tucked in. The head needs to be kept erect, as if a string were attached to the top, pulling it up. Please remember all of this important knowledge. Your spinal alignment will sustain your internal energy flow.

Dr. Maoshing Ni: What my father says is true. If the body's posture and alignment are poor, the flow of *chi* becomes blocked and defeats the whole purpose of gentle movement. The important thing to remember when you learn good posture is to practice it at every moment of your life.

D. Center of Gravity

Master Ni: The mid point of the human body is the Lower *Tan Tien,* which is located just below the navel. This should be your center of gravity, the place from which your movements originate when practicing most *chi* exercises. The three *Tan Tien* are also called the Three Origins.

The movements of *T'ai Chi* are done in a standing position, thus it has a different requirement and purpose than sitting cultivation. Sitting meditation has its center of gravity in the Middle *Tan Tien,* the heart area. Keeping your center in the Lower *Tan Tien* strengthens both your physical and sexual stamina. However, please do not practice *T'ai Chi* movement just to increase your sexual pleasure. Do it for your health.

Sexual strength is the source of physical health and longevity. A person whose sexual energy dies off at an early age cannot live to be very old. Do not rush into lots of sexual activity; not because you do not have the desire for it, but so that you can guard that energy and use it throughout your life. The sexual energy generated by *T'ai Chi* movement improves your internal circulation and enhances all aspects of your life.

E. Gracefulness of Body and Spirit

Master Ni: The word "graceful" is generally used as an adjective, but it can be more than just a word in the dictionary, it can be a description of your life. You can cultivate gracefulness by practicing any of the forms of *Chi Kung (Chi Gong)* and *T'ai Chi.*

No force is used in practicing gentle *chi* exercises. *Chi* moves, *chi* speaks and *chi* sings a natural, sweet and happy melody. You can express its melody of natural transformation through your movements and your life.

Dr. Maoshing Ni: Try to do all your movements in a gentle manner. Do not thrash around. Relax. It is a gentle process of moving *chi* through the body. If you do anything abruptly, you can block the flow and end up with a headache or some other discomfort.

F. Evenness and Fullness

Master Ni: There is a special requirement called *jung yun yuan*

mang 均匀圓滿

Jung yun means evenness, with nothing sticking out, nothing unusual. Even if you place special emphasis on a certain movement, that movement will not "stick out" to an external observer.

Yuan mang means fullness. To be full means the whole body, from the *Tan Tien* to the finger, from the soles of your feet even to the tip of your hair, is full of energy.

Together, the phrase means that full development is attained through movement.

G. After You Practice

After you finish your practice, if you are young, your stomach makes noise and wants something to eat. Slowly enjoy your meal, and do not eat too much. In the evening, before they go to bed, young people might have some body heat from food that has not been burned off and is still in the head. This makes it hard to fall asleep. Practicing Cosmic Tour at that time will make you sleep a "thousand-year sleep," and the next day you will wake up refreshed and ready to start another day.

Q: What sort of diet is most beneficial for practicing T'ai Chi?

Master Ni: A light one, both in quality and quantity. Don't eat too much bread or rice or other heavy foods. Serious *chi* students usually eat very light foods like Chinese porridge, which is also called rice soup. It is easily digested, so you have time to do *T'ai Chi* again. If you eat regular foods until you have a full belly, it will take four hours to digest it and you will not have time to do *T'ai Chi* any more, because then it is time for your next meal. Instead, eat light foods in small amounts. This will be beneficial to your practice.

Sometimes I feel I eat too much, because I enjoy gourmet food, but it is too difficult to do *T'ai Chi* if you are interested in gourmet food. If you are really devoted to *T'ai Chi*, maybe you can keep one day a month to enjoy gourmet food during a certain season. However, whether you eat simple food or gourmet food, do not practice *T'ai Chi* on a full stomach.

Section 3: Principles of Practice

Master Ni: Some of the important principles of movement apply to daily life as well. Once you understand and learn to follow these principles, you will see how natural and how much more comfortable they are than abrupt, rough or violent movements. They will help you become more naturally productive, creative and supportive. You will begin to notice how each movement of your *T'ai Chi* practice or each action in your life naturally produces the next one, which creates the next, so that each supports the other.

The following adaptations of traditional *T'ai Chi* movement classics elucidate the practice of this art (reprinted from *Tao, the Subtle Universal Law)*:

> T'ai Chi, the ultimate form, arises out of *wu chi*, the Undivided Oneness. It is the origin of movement and stillness, and the Mother of yin and yang. In movement it generates, in stillness it returns. Neither exceeding nor falling short, *T'ai Chi* moves in bending and stretching. When one yields to a hard force, this is called 'moving around it.' When one tackles a hard force, this is called 'sticking with it.'
>
> When the other's movement comes quickly, respond quickly. When the other's movement comes slowly, follow slowly. In the myriad changing situations, this principle stays the same.
>
> From familiarity with the exercise comes a gradual realization and understanding of energy. From the understanding of energy there comes spiritual illumination. Yet only after long, diligent practice will this sudden clarity be achieved.
>
> Empty and alert, still and quiet. The breath sinks into the Lower *Tan Tien*. Not inclined, not leaning. Suddenly concealing, suddenly manifesting. When an intruding weight comes to my left, my left is empty. When an intruding weight comes to my right, then my right disappears.
>
> Looking up, the other feels my height. Looking down, the other feels my depth. Advancing, he feels the distance lengthening. Retreating, he is more crowded. A small bird cannot take off, because there is no solid part to ascend from. Nor can a single fly land. The opponent does not know where the energy is changing in me, but I alone know where the opponent's force is located.
>
> When great heroes are without match, it is because of all of these factors. There are many other techniques of combat. Whatever their differences, they all nevertheless rely on the

strong to overcome the weak, and the slow to give in to the fast. Yet as far as the strong beating the weak, the slow giving in to the fast, such things derive from natural abilities and do not have to be studied. When 'four ounces move a thousand pounds' it is obviously not a matter of strength. When an old man can withstand many young men, how can it be a matter of speed?

Stand as poised as a scale. In action be like a wheel. With the center of your gravity displaced to one side, you can be fluid. If you are 'double heavy,' with your weight evenly distributed on both feet, you become stagnant. Often one encounters someone who, even after many years of study, has not achieved proper development and is still subdued by others. This is because he has not realized the fault of 'double heaviness.' To avoid this fault, one must know yin and yang. To stick is also to move away and to move away is also to stick. *Yin* does not leave *yang* and *yang* does not leave *yin*. *Yin* and *yang* always complement each other. It is necessary to understand this in order to understand energy. With an understanding of energy, the more one practices, the more wonderful will be one's development. One comprehends in silence and experiences in feeling, until gradually one may act at will.

The traditional advice to deny self and to yield to the other has been misunderstood to mean one should abandon the near and seek the far. Only a true Master has the skill to demonstrate this principle. A mistake of inches, but an error of a thousand leagues. Therefore, the student needs to pay careful heed to what is said.

The above was adapted from *The Treatise on T'ai Chi Chuan*, attributed to Wang, Chung-Yueh, the foremost pupil of Tsan, San Fong.

The following is adapted from *A Discussion of the Practice of T'ai Chi Ch'uan*, a traditional text that is sometimes attributed to Master Tsan, San Fong who lived in the 13th century:

When one begins to move, the entire body should be light and flexible, and the movement must be continuous. The chi should be expanded with vitality and the mind should be kept tranquil. Do not allow gaps, unevenness or discontinuities. Your feet are the root of energy, which passes through the legs, is controlled by the waist, and finally emerges through the fingers. Your feet, legs and waist need to be coordinated so that in moving forward and backward you have good control of time and space. Without this control of time and space in all movements - up, down, left, right, forward and backward - your body will be in disorder and the fault must be sought in the waist and legs. All of these principles concern the will rather than what is external.

When there is up, there must be down; when there is left, there must be right. The will to go up implies the will to go down. For if upon lifting an opposing force you add the idea of pushing it down, then the root of your opposition is broken and without doubt you will overcome it quickly.

The empty and the solid can be clearly distinguished. Every physical situation by nature has an empty side and a solid side. Let there be continuity in the movements of the entire body. Let there be not the slightest break.

The mind moves the chi calmly and naturally, directing it deeply inward; then it can be gathered into the bones and marrow. The chi moves the entire being smoothly and continuously; then the form can easily follow the mind. If your energies are vitalized, then there is no problem about being sluggish and heavy. To accomplish this the spine needs to be erect as if the head were suspended. The mind and chi must move flexibly in order to achieve smoothness and roundness of movement. This is accomplished by the interchange of yin and yang.

To concentrate the energy one must sink one's center of gravity, maintain looseness and quietude, and focus one's energy in a single direction. To stand, one must remain centrally poised, calm and expanded; one can thus protect himself from all sides. Move the energy as delicately as a string of pearls, so there is no place that it does not reach. Refine your essence to become as flawless as steel so there is no obstruction it cannot destroy.

One's appearance is like that of a hawk catching a rabbit; one's spirit, like a cat watching a mouse. In rest, be as still as a mountain; in movement, like a river. Store the energy as if drawing a bow. Issue the energy as if releasing the arrow.

Through the curve seek the straight. First store, then release. The energy issues from the spine. Steps follow changes in the form. To withdraw is to release. To release is to withdraw. To break is to continue. Back and forth must have folds, no straight path in either case, in order to prepare and gather the energy. Advancing and retreating must have turns and changes.

Through what is greatly soft one achieves what is greatly strong. If one is able to inhale and exhale, then one can be light and flexible. Breathing must be nourished without impediment, no holding of the breath and no forcing it; then no harm will come. The energy must be bent like a bow and stored, then you will always have more than you need. When the mind orders, the *chi* goes forth as a banner, and the waist takes the command. First seek to stretch and expand; afterwards seek to tighten and collect; then one attains integrated development.

It is said: first the mind, afterwards the body. The abdomen is relaxed, the *chi* is gathered into the bones, the spirit is at ease and the body quiet. Be totally conscious at every moment.

It must be remembered:

As one part moves, all parts move; if one part is still, all parts are still. Pull and move, go and come, the chi goes to the back and is gathered in the spine, making the spirit firm and leisurely manifesting calm without. Step as a cat walks. Use force as if pulling silk. Throughout the body, concentrate on the spirit, not on the *chi*. To concentrate on the *chi* causes stagnation. To be with *chi*, or holding the breath, is to be without strength. To be without *chi*, moving the breath and allowing it to flow freely, one can be really strong. The breath is like a cart's wheel. The waist is like its axle.

(adapted from the *Essential Principles for Practicing T'ai Chi Ch'uan*, by W.S. Wu, 1812-1880)

A. The *T'ai Chi* Principle

The cosmic *t'ai chi* principle is that of rhythmic alternation or movement. For example, inhaling and exhaling, or moving inward to collect energy in the center before moving outward from the center to the limbs. Most of you already understand the concept of *yin* and *yang* as the two poles of all things. The cosmic *t'ai chi* principle is simply the alternation of these two forces.

The special term for the *t'ai chi* principle is *yin yang kai huh*. *Yin* and *yang* can be translated as contraction and expansion. *Kai* means openness and *huh* means to close back. Thus, *kai huh* actually means the same thing as *yin yang*.

If you learn the principle of *yin yang kai huh*, then you know the most important guideline for how to do things and how to apply your strength or mind in all aspects of life, including business. Everything follows a pattern of rhythmic alternation. There is so much theory about this, but the reality never changes.

More interesting than talking or reading about the theory is experiencing the reality by practicing these ancient movements which have been developed and refined by generations of devoted practitioners. Doing them will broaden your understanding more than reading ten thousand books. They are all gentle movements, but the energy of each is quite different.

B. Naturalness

Master Ni: In all your movements, whether as exercise or in daily life activities, the key to success ·is naturalness. Nothing about these exercises is artificial or superficial. They are all deeply related to your natural physiological structure and how your energy flows through that structure.

Each movement of *T'ai Chi* describes a circle. There are no abrupt or radical changes in direction, speed or style. You just keep making circles: small ones, large ones, horizontal, vertical or slanted ones, in all directions. All movements can be considered as one movement, because they are connected. Whether you reach out or gather back, the pattern is cyclical. Some circles are too small to observe, but energywise they are a whirlpool.

The ancient achieved ones learned that there is no way that we can fight our own nature. For example, can you use your ear as a mouth to eat? No, you cannot. Can you use your eye to breathe? No, you cannot. Nature is nature. You have to learn to be compliant with nature regarding the basics. No one needs to think about being natural. Even without the conscious mind, the body responds harmoniously to most situations.

We cannot go against the nature of the universe. For example, if you sow seeds in winter with the intent of harvesting in spring, nothing will grow. Today, people use greenhouses, and by controlling light, temperature and water they can make things grow. Nevertheless, even greenhouses are subject to natural limitations.

The ancient, gentle exercises illustrate cosmic principles and can bring one into great harmony with cosmic law as they guide and conduct one's internal energy. Cosmic law is important for personal internal harmonization, because each individual life is a small model of the universe.

The original gentle *chi* exercises are the result of the spiritual achievement and natural minds of sages who wished to maintain the wholeness of their spirit. *T'ai Chi* movement is a natural movement that imitates the stars and galaxies that move around us and the internal movement inside each life. Today these same exercises can still help people return to naturalness.

C. Be Simple

Master Ni: Simplicity is important in spiritual cultivation. You might think that *T'ai Chi* movement is not simple, but it teaches you to govern complexity with simplicity. The Way also teaches you to govern complex situations with the refined simplicity of your spirit. The principle of simplicity can be learned by doing *T'ai Chi* movement, but it is not *T'ai Chi* movement. The principle of simplicity can be applied to all situations in your life and business. A big company, a big government and the world itself can be understood and managed by simplicity. Simplicity is effective. If you engage in complications, you lose yourself. Learn to be simple.

D. Be Gentle

Master Ni: It is important to learn to be gentle and non-violent in speech, thought, emotion or action. Wise people know that treating others violently is the same as treating themselves violently. In *T'ai Chi* movement, you can learn to be gentle. To be simple and gentle in daily life is one manifestation of the Integral Truth.

E. Be Unassertive and Non-Dominating

Master Ni: Be unassertive and non-dominating. Reality is always in the process of change. You only need to respond correctly to a changing situation. No situation is static, so no prearranged response will be effective. Ordinary people have preconceptions about life having to be a certain way, so they become nervous and act prematurely, which only makes the situation worse and causes real damage to other people and themselves.

F. Be Balanced and Poised

Master Ni: The next principle is to be balanced and poised in movement. You might think that is easy, but I don't think so. For example, even if a person sits still, is he calm and poised? Many people cannot even sit still. In *T'ai Chi* movement, you learn the principle of balance and poise.

G. Be Calm

Master Ni: Learn to be calm, especially in rough situations. The flow of *T'ai Chi* movement is calm. Most *Chi Kung (Chi Gong)* movements also follow this principle. Some styles of *Chi Kung (Chi Gong)* or martial arts may be vigorous, but a violent force never lasts for long.

H. Be Kind to All

Master Ni: Be kind to all beings. *T'ai Chi* movement is not damaging or harmful in any way.

I. Be Clear In Mind

Master Ni: Develop mental clarity and do not emphasize individual movements. *T'ai Chi* is an integral set of movements that are not discrete. It requires smoothness and completeness to weave all the pieces together in a integral whole.

J. Be Frugal

Master Ni: The principle of frugality relates to daily life as much as to *chi* exercise. It is important to be frugal with regard to attachment to material objects, but abundant in gathering your energy. Both in daily life and in *chi* practice, you should protect your vital force and be frugal in using it. Do not be overly confident in using your physical, material and mental strength, but be prepared and make your practice a great source of energy provision for yourself. Be unattached to victory. Be frugal in the use of energy. Be rich in energy preparation or gathering. Make sure you always have enough energy to handle all situations.

Learn from gentle *chi* exercise and from the *yin/yang* principle (the cosmic *t'ai chi* principle) how to use your life force in a rhythmic pattern. *Yin* and *yang* means there is day and night in which you experience movement and quietness. If your hand stretches out, you must draw it back. If you kick your leg high, it must come down. Before you can jump high, you must first learn to crawl. If there is a left side, there must be a right side. If you have a front, you must have a back. You must take care of the whole thing, not just go forward without ever retreating, or walk to the left and never go right. Alternation and rhythmic movement are the principle of *yin* and *yang*. Do not overextend yourself in any of the *T'ai Chi* movements or in anything you do in your life. Be frugal with your energy, and use this helpful principle in your daily life.

K. Know Where to Use Energy

Master Ni: Another principle of *T'ai Chi* practice is to know the right time and place to use your energy so that your strength is applied efficiently to activities that are righteous and just.

This brings us to the next principle, which is smoothly avoiding a possible confrontation. Be unwilling to proceed with foolish action. *T'ai Chi* movement never confronts force; you always yield. In daily life, this means not seeking profit or gain for unworthy or evil purposes. The purpose of this yielding is not to yield just for the sake of yielding, but to avoid confrontation and still be a winner.

Section 4: Advanced Practice

A. Deepening Your Practice

Master Ni: Practically speaking, the dissolution of the personal self requires devotion. When you begin to learn the form, you must do it correctly. Once you know the form, you can go much deeper with your practice.

The external form is the first level to achieve. To reach true mastery, you must continue to practice until it is not you doing the movement. Then, you continue to practice the movement until your entire life and everything you do merge with the cosmic law and there is no personal self. It takes many years to reach this level, but it is well worth the effort. From the relative movement of *yin* and *yang*, the polarized energies, you find the absolute.

The art of gentle movement is very personal, and some people never let others observe them doing it, because it is their personal treasure. A few share it with others.

At the same time that you learn the practice, it is important to understand spiritual self-cultivation, to study general energy channels from acupuncture books, and so forth. You do not necessarily need to become an expert, but all the knowledge you obtain supports your learning. It is important to not stay on the surface but go deeper, beyond the movement and the physics. If you learn this, you will experience gentle movement as a kind of self-discovery and discovery of nature. If you practice it regularly, you will achieve many things that cannot be described in words.

B. Switch Sides Practice

Master Ni: We are all born with a natural tendency to be either right-handed or left-handed. The habit of using one side of the body too much in daily activities, while the other side does nothing, creates or aggravates an imbalance. In order to correct such imbalanced development, *chi* practice offers an opportunity to use both sides of the body.

For example, I am right-handed. When I was small, I could not successfully use my left hand to cut the fingernails of my right hand with scissors. My mother suggested that I overcome this shortcoming, so on many occasions, I switched hands when doing things. I learned *T'ai Chi* movement on the right side, as everybody does, but in my personal practice, I reverse the movements and do it also on the left. I usually practice the left more than the right, because I already use my right limbs a lot in daily life. Reversing the right movements and doing them on the left side is not all that difficult to do.

Generally, people have more strength on one side than on the other. That seems to be a natural arrangement that cannot be considered a problem. However, I do it just to give myself a small challenge and because I do not wish my left side to become too clumsy.

C. A Different Way to Organize Your Practice

Master Ni: When I have time, I do the art starting with the left side on odd days and the right side on even days. Or, I do the left ones in the morning and the right ones in the afternoon, or vice versa. If I have a whole hour for practice, first I do Gentle Path because it is slow, then I do Sky Journey because it picks up the energy and is faster. I then finish with Infinite Expansion as a peak to generate internal and external energy. It takes almost 40 minutes for me to do all three. Afterward, I slow down to collect my energy back to normalcy.

This arrangement is only one suggestion or possibility. Practicing the physical arts should always be done flexibly and should never push you. It needs to be adjusted to suit your daily activities and stage of life.

D. Evolving to Self-Guidance

Master Ni: *T'ai Chi* Exercise, as I teach it, has a pure spiritual purpose: for maintaining internal and external unity. Even after years and years of practice, you will never become tired of it. Although I do different forms, they are all the great companions of my life. Some are suitable to do in certain types of weather, different seasons, days, and hours. When you become achieved, you will know what movements are most suitable for certain times and conditions.

All internal movement is adjustable, depending on your knowledge about yourself. You are not fixed by the form. From reading and from your own achieved spiritual knowledge, you can learn to guide yourself for maximum benefit. Eventually, self-guidance becomes necessary for all who use physical movement to achieve spiritual development.

E. Special Enjoyment

Master Ni: When I have a chance, I sometimes practice physical arts with harmonious music in a beautiful garden with a sweet breeze and the chirping of birds. The trophy I win is filling my life with pleasure and joy.

Chapter Conclusion

Master Ni: Meditation or *chi* movement like *T'ai Chi* does not involve deep thinking. However, a certain level of understanding can provide a good foundation for such arts. I have already recommended reading the *Tao Teh Ching*. The words *Tao Teh Ching*, or "guidance for the direction of universal morality and virtue," mean the same thing as *wu wei*, which is usually translated as "do nothing extra." *Wu wei* means that in meditation, your mind does not long for anything. It has, and you have, no ambition. Do not be ambitious about your meditation or your cultivation; that would disturb your mind. Do not hold any kind of worry or fear about anything. Do not be partial to anything else. For example, if you sit there and you think "I would like to see Buddha, I would like to see the Holy Mother," that is being partial.

T'ai Chi movement is part of the direct path. On the direct path, people have no need for external religion, because personal spiritual truth is what the person is and does. External religion often involves conceptual duality or dependence on a final judgement from someone else. This can cause problems in one's life and development. The direct path transcends religious beliefs. All faiths, when they reach the non-conceptual level, embody the integral truth.

People with truthful attitudes are always seeking to improve themselves. The language of each region in the world may be different, but the purpose of all languages is to serve the substance of life. Likewise, the purpose of all rituals and ceremonies is enlightenment. People may arrive at the mountain top from different directions, but once they are at the top, they all enjoy the same panoramic view.

In daily life, we like to be able to be receptive, flexible, impartial, mature, responsible, responsive, and non-glaring. Non-glare is like a translucent glass or mirror instead of a direct, blinding light. The martial arts can show off a person's talent or physical force, but in *T'ai Chi* movement and in a spiritual life, we prefer to be non-glaring. There is a proverb here in the West that says, "Everything that glitters is not gold." In its natural state, gold ore does not shine, but there is a glittery mineral called "Fool's Gold." We could also say that we like to be "non-glittery."

Your spiritual achievement depends on what you do, your level of understanding, how much you delve into it, and how much you receive from the achievement. Although there are different levels of spiritual achievement, can you ever decide that what you have achieved is completely true and final? Spiritual achievement is the unending personal opportunity to reach the ultimate truth. In spirit as well as body, therefore, the same basic principle applies: keep moving.

Chapter 5

Poem for Reaching Infinity

A Life of Infinity

A world of vastness and emptiness:
the deep mountain.
There lives a life of infinity
with no company,
no worldly communication.

You enjoy the set of movements.
This is your cultivation.
This is your achievement.
This is your enlightenment.
This is your merit.
The movement unites your form with your shadow,
your mind with your will.
The surroundings become quiet and join your movement.
With this movement,
you surpass your life and death.
The years and centuries melt away.
All dissolves into nothing.

The twilight of morning and the light of the moon
accompany you
in smashing the white cloud to pieces.
It is transformed into dew,
bringing moisture to lives everywhere.
Your movement is inaudible,
yet it has a gentle rhythm.
It is like playing, singing and chanting:
"Holy, Holy, and Holy!"
You continue the work of creation of all gods.
You span the bridge of eternity
between existence and non-existence,
ego and non-ego.
With no language and no posture,
but using the language above all languages
and the movement above all movements,
you link the past of no beginning
and the future of no end.
You leave no trace or seam
in the perfect welding of these two
in integral oneness.

99

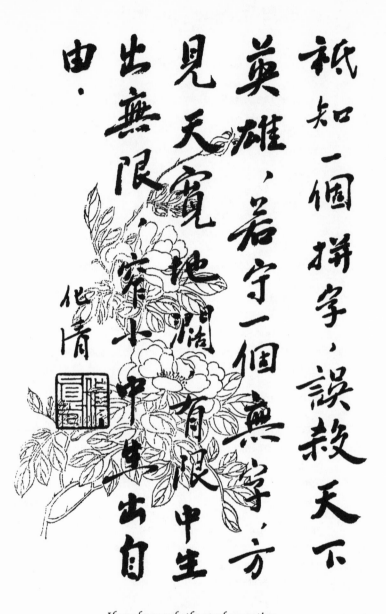

祇知一個拼字，誤救天下
英雄，若守一個無字，方
見天寬地闊，有限中生
出無限，窄小中生出自
由。

化清

If you learn only the word competing,
  you have wronged the meaning of hero.
If you also know the word nothing,
  the world is so big to you.
Thus, you will experience moving from limitation
  to attain unlimitedness,
  and from the narrow world,
  you attain freedom.

Chapter 6

The Basis of Physical Arts: *Chi*

From familiarity with the exercise comes a gradual realization and understanding of energy. From the understanding of energy comes spiritual illumination, yet only after long, diligent practice will this sudden breakthrough be achieved.

- Wang, Chung-Yueh, the foremost pupil of Tsan, San Fong

Q: What is energy or chi?

Master Ni: The energy that the ancient developed ones called *chi* is nothing other than nature. More accurately speaking, nature is a flow of energy that is constantly forming and reforming as time and space. People can see water flow, but they do not see the flow of the entire world and themselves with it. You can decide whether to be in or out of the flow.

Most people think a good life means enjoying leisure and not moving, but that is not a good life, that is stagnation. A negative attitude toward life goes against nature. A person who is aware of and goes with the flow of nature and normalcy is not stuck psychologically. Moving and flowing is the key to life and to learning the Universal Integral Way.

Because water is so common and visible, it provides a good model for understanding the movement of life. Good water, like a good life, is not stagnant or polluted because it keeps flowing. Stagnation causes life to decay and die. This principle also applies to your emotions.

The physical exercise or *chi* exercise described in this book is the art of moving *chi* through the body. All life movement is related to *chi;* however, there are different levels or depths which can be experienced or known.

Dr. Maoshing Ni: It is *chi* that allows us to go about our daily lives. People without enough *chi* can barely get through the day. By the time the day ends, they are exhausted, not just mentally, but physically and spiritually as well.

Many attempts have been made to explain the general and specific nature of *chi,* however none can ever completely encompass the reality. *Chi* might be considered the "invisible fuel" or driving force behind every living and functioning thing. *Chi* is heat, light, color, electromagnetic fields, radiation, etc. In its broadest definition, *chi* or energy is everything, including movement exhibiting frequency or waves.

About 25 years ago, scientific research began to study *chi* in the human body. There have been attempts to measure the *chi* coming out of the hands of *Chi Kung (Chi Gong)* practitioners. Scientific instruments were able to detect components like heat, light, near infrared frequencies, electromagnetic fields and other micro-particles in what is referred to as *chi*.

There are two main components or qualities to *chi*. One is the substantial or physical aspect, which can be measured. This can be felt as heat, tingling, crawling (like a little bug crawling up your arm) when you do *chi* exercise. The other is insubstantial. This is the aspect that carries or transmits information throughout the body.

Traditional Chinese Medicine understands that the mind is not synonymous with the brain. Each individual cell of the body has its own intelligence. The mind is controlled through the spirit, which is housed in the heart, and every cell in our body is monitored or communicated with through *chi*. There is a definite informational quality to *chi*, a message that is communicated to your body. That means if I conceive the thought "I am going to heal my sprained ankle," and I continue to think or send the message, thought or visualization to that part of my body, healing occurs.

Master Ni: I accept the hidden potential of *chi* as reality. For example, many years ago, shops and houses in Chinese towns were built one right next to the other. The buildings were mostly wood, so if one building caught on fire, the rest would quickly burn also.

Once there was a fire in a neighborhood in which there was a shopkeeper who had an iron safe in his office. The ancient safe, which was made of iron and was very heavy, contained all his money and valuables. On this occasion, he picked the safe up and moved it outside to a place he considered was far enough away from the fire. After the fire was over and his shop was no longer endangered, he needed to move the iron safe back inside, but he this time he had to hire a team of people to move it. Everyone asked him, "How could you have done that by yourself?" and he didn't know how he could have possibly moved something so heavy.

When there is an emergency, if a person's inner power is complete, they can do many things that they are unable to do in normal life. Great subtle power is stored as natural potential in your life, unless you damage it.

Q: Is chi *something I experience in my everyday life and am not aware of?*

Master Ni: When your internal energy is enhanced, improved or increased, you feel lighter. When it is full, you feel that you can handle things much more easily and confidently, and you are not as nervous. When it is too full, like a healthy 17 year old's, you had better use it in a positive direction such as *chi* exercise. When your internal energy is low, or your head is congested from over-sleeping, you feel irritable.

The small situations in life can help you learn to understand your internal situation, become more aware of it, and eventually manage it.

Q: You mentioned that if someone oversleeps he will feel sluggish or congested. What can a person do to remedy that?

Master Ni: Do the first four sections of the Eight Treasures. If you oversleep, you need to take longer to adjust yourself. What happens is that your muscles have less oxygen and become acidified. That toxic condition gathers and becomes stagnant inside. This is especially true for people who are in the habit of eating a big evening meal. Lack of activity in the evening means the food is not totally digested and absorbed by the body. This also creates a toxic condition. Over the long term, an accumulation of such toxicity will give you trouble.

The amount of sleep you get is important. Do not make a habit of looking for excitement and stimulation before going to sleep, or you won't have a sound, restful sleep. Such stimulation and the resulting poor sleep will make it difficult to wake up the next morning, because you have no strength. Repeating this habit starts a vicious cycle that will only get worse: stimulation before sleep, a disturbed system, no strength in the morning, rising late, and having your entire system dulled by the loss of the morning hours that can refresh you.

Thus, you need to watch your eating and sleeping habits. In the morning work vigorously, and in the evening avoid stimulation. This is what I learned, but it is not usually what modern people like to do.

To practice any form of *chi kung (chi gong)* without taking a good look at diet, lifestyle, sexual activity, etc., is like going on a "chocolate diet." There is no benefit. The best results from doing *chi* exercise are seen when one develops a consistently healthy, normal lifestyle.

Dr. Maoshing Ni: *Chi Kung (Chi Gong)* is a mental and physical method that enables human beings to acquire skill or strength through working with the body's bioenergy. *Chi* and *Chi Kung (Chi Gong)* are the basis of acupuncture, Traditional Chinese Medicine, and many styles of martial arts. One of the most attractive features of *Chi Kung (Chi Gong)* is its effectiveness in health maintenance and in self-healing of many chronic conditions. A well-trained *Chi Kung (Chi Gong)* practitioner can also utilize the bio-energy called *chi* to treat patients.

In history, *Chi Kung (Chi Gong)* was a popular activity in China. It was practiced within families, by monks, spiritual people, martial artists, and many people in the field of Traditional Chinese Medicine.

Q: What exactly is chi *exercise?*

Dr. Daoshing Ni: *Chi Kung (Chi Gong)* is a set of exercises practiced in such a way as to regulate and recover the circulation of *chi* in the body and to strengthen the processes and ability of self-healing. *Chi* is the underlying "substance" responsible for health and sickness. Exercise, and a way of life that strengthens this vital energy, are what the ancient developed ones believed to be the keys to immortality.

Chi Kung (Chi Gong) may seem very "mystical" or "new-age" to Western culture, but it has been around for thousands of years and is not hard to learn. To the beginning student, the first "sensation" of the flow of *chi* is an exciting experience. This is usually a "pins and needles" effect that emerges at various points in the hands, because this is the easiest place to "touch" the *chi*. After this, one begins to feel the *chi* flow through various channels and unblock various acupuncture points, sometimes causing spontaneous movement of the limbs. This is the so-called "Alpha" state in psychology, accompanied by feelings of being energized, spirited, and relaxed. Mental stress and physical tension are greatly reduced, bringing about an overall feeling of peacefulness and relaxation.

Crane-Style *Chi Gong* is becoming increasingly popular, because it is easy to learn and the flow of *chi* is more easily felt than in many other styles. The Crane Style is also especially noted for having excellent benefits in people with chronic disorders. After three months of consistent practice, one can usually start to feel the activation of the *chi* at a specific point of the body. It takes longer, obviously, to be able to feel the flow of *chi* throughout the complete system of channels.

Q: Why is it helpful to do exercises that stimulate chi?

Master Ni: There are several levels or reasons why one may desire to do any kind of *chi* practice or *chi* exercise, which will be described by my son Maoshing.

Dr. Maoshing Ni: One level is simply for health and disease prevention. *Chi* exercises are different from conventional exercise in that there is a component of healing that takes place. Although regular exercise is good as a health maintenance program, it is not specifically therapeutic.

For example, scientists have documented certain healing phenomena that occur as a result of regular *chi* exercise. One of these is the enhancement of the immune system. There is an increase in production of T-helper cells and white blood cells when *chi* practice is performed for 45 minutes to an hour. There is also an increased flow of blood throughout the body, especially in the micro-capillaries. This improves the transportation of waste products out of and nutrients and oxygen into the cells of the body.

When *Chi Kung (Chi Gong)* or *chi* exercise is practiced on a regular basis, there is also a regulating effect on the hormonal system of various glandular activities. There is also a normalization of the nervous system, especially the autonomic nervous system. These scientific studies provide evidence that there are definite physical benefits to practicing *chi* exercise.

A second level is that of self-mastery. *Chi* exercise can help refine your emotions. It is difficult to become overly emotional when you are calm and composed after a session of *chi* exercise, so it is a great tranquilizer for the mind, and is thus effective in dealing with stress. With regular practice, your memory will improve and your mind will become sharper. Through such improved mental acuity, your performance in every aspect of life correspondingly improves.

You can develop your own innate power through the practice of *chi*. Some *Chi Kung (Chi Gong)* practitioners develop seemingly supernatural powers such as the ability to sense which part of a person is diseased. They also develop a sensitivity to negative changes in their own body, other people's bodies and the environment. Expert practitioners are also able to develop healing capabilities with their *chi*.

This *chi* we are talking about can be explained in many different ways. One simple example is to presume that the body is a battery with negative and positive charges and different chemicals that constantly generate nerve impulses. A diseased person is similar to a worn-out battery. For that person, the *chi* healer would be able to affect the quality and the quantity of *chi* or energy in the body and thereby normalize the electromagnetic fields. When the battery is normalized and recharged, so to speak, there will be recovery from the imbalance.

The human body is extremely intricate, and there are many environmental changes and influences that can throw it off. Hence there is a constant effort to strive for equilibrium.

Serious *chi* practitioners often strive for a third level of practice, that of mind control. In recent years, an abundance of research has been done in the area of body/mind connection and how the mind can affect the functions of the body.

Q: What should I do to make my practice more like chi *exercise rather than just physical exercise?*

Dr. Maoshing Ni: When practicing, and at all times in your daily life as well, keep your tongue curled up against the roof of your mouth. This connects two important channels in this area. The Conception *(Ren)* Channel runs through the front midline of the body to the bottom of the tongue. The Governing (*Du*) Channel runs up the center line of the back, along the spine and over the top of the head to the roof of your mouth. When the tongue curls up, so that the bottom of the tongue is touching the roof of the mouth, it makes a bridge that allows the flow of *chi* to be continuous. This is important.

In the beginning, you can visualize this flow of *chi* as warm water flowing through the channels in your body and feel the sensations as you visualize it. After a while, as you become more proficient in your practice and mastery of *chi*, you will feel the *chi* without much visualization. Then you can simply guide the flow. Once you are even more proficient, the *chi* will flow naturally, by itself, in the right pathways without guidance.

Q: Is there such a thing as good chi *and bad* chi*? Some spiritual teachings promote that there is only one energy, and that it is basically benevolent.*

Master Ni: Energy is all around us. To refer to "good *chi*" or "bad *chi*" is to talk about the *chi* in people's bodies or the environment. Some people have a lot of life energy, and you feel good when you are around them. It is the same for a good place, but people are usually less aware of that.

"Bad *chi*" usually describes an energy blockage or mental disorientation. So there is such a thing as good energy or bad energy, but people's lives can be improved by spiritual cultivation. This is what my teaching is all about.

Dr. Maoshing Ni: *Chi* exercise is a way to rid your body of unhealthy, negative energy. The human body is a receptacle of all kinds of energy. We absorb *chi* all the time and must be careful about what we take in. This is a conscious awareness that we must develop. Eliminating turbid *chi* from the body is like taking an internal shower everyday.

Your focus needs to be on strengthening yourself and improving and refining your *chi* so that it becomes good *chi*. In other words, we want more good *chi* and less bad *chi*. It helps to live in an environment that is supportive and positive, to take in good *chi* via a good diet, to be careful, and to expose oneself to positive elements that give off good *chi* such as trees, mountains, pristine lakes, good air, forests, fresh air, etc.

Everyone can take precautions to avoid bad *chi*. It is obvious that walking behind a car or bus and breathing the exhaust, or exposing oneself to other types of pollution, is not wise. There are places that have a concentration of negative energy. If you are sensitive, you can avoid such places. Some are obvious, such as bars or nightclubs full of smoke and loud disturbing music, but some are not. The sources and consequences of bad *chi* can some-times be quite subtle. Bad *chi* can be as simple as someone being angry, agitated or aggressive.

Wise people avoid exposing themselves to bad *chi*, and at the same time focus on refining and uplifting their personal energy. Good *chi* can be generated by positive thoughts. Conversely, bad *chi* will result from negative thoughts or emotions.

Q: If you are saying that we receive chi *from all things around us, then what are the sources of good or beneficial* chi?

Master Ni: Your health, well-being, psychology and capability are affected by the energy of your environment. This becomes the focus of architecture, interior design, fashion, landscaping, etc. All of these things can support your happiness and productivity. The most inexpensive way is to be simple and bright in living and in how you use things.

Q: How does chi *actually move?*

Dr. Maoshing Ni: Within and around the body, we have channels, sometimes called meridians, in which *chi* flows. These channels cannot be seen, but they can be measured by skin resistance tests. We can feel them and we can send *chi* through them by conscious effort, thereby initiating a healing, strengthening or reinforcing process.

The body stores *chi* in the *Tan Tien*. When practicing *Chi Kung (Chi Gong)*, you take your *chi* out of the *Tan Tien* to circulate it, then you bring it back into the *Tan Tien*.

Q: When I practice chi *exercises, will I feel or experience anything unusual?*

Master Ni: One of Maoshing's students can explain what she has learned from attending classes of *chi* exercise and her own experience in practice and teaching others.

Student: Some people experience the sensation of *chi,* either during *chi* exercise or during meditation, as a feeling of coldness, aching or heaviness, tingling, warmth or a crawling sensation on the skin. Sometimes there will be a slight shaking or moving of a limb or the body. That is okay, because it means that the *chi* from inside is starting to surface.

If a part of your body, such as your leg, feels heavy, it means that *chi* is trapped there. To move it out, you simply shake your leg. If you experience a sensation of tingling at the bottom of your feet, that is good because it means the *chi* has arrived there.

When you do some *chi* exercises, you may start to feel a little flushed or your body may become hot. Do not worry about it, just keep doing it.

Dr. Maoshing Ni: Sometimes an overwhelming emotion may suddenly come up and then pass. When slight dizziness, minor swelling or mild pain occurs anywhere in the body as you exercise, it means that your body is attempting to move the *chi* through potential blockages. If you get dizzy, just sit down. If palpitation or shortness of breath occurs, it just means that the *chi* is going through blockages in the body.

When you practice *Chi Kung (Chi Gong)*, do not pay too much attention to the sensations that go on in your body. Just continue to practice, try to keep your mind focused, and keep moving the *chi.*

During meditation, if involuntary or automatic movements occur, let the body (trunk, legs, arms and/or hands) move in the direction it naturally wants to go, but continue to maintain the preparatory breath with the movements. The body movements are a result of the body's natural adjustment/aligning process.

Q: On the whole, how should we manage our energy in our daily life?

Master Ni: Energy is like money, and how you manage your energy is often similar to how you manage your money. Life energy is even more valuable than money, so you should learn to use it correctly and effectively. It can be put to good use in your own life and in the lives of other people whom you choose to help. Use it wisely.

Q: If someone does an exercise that builds strong muscles, will that affect their practice of T'ai Chi?

Master Ni: Tight muscles will affect your *T'ai Chi* practice negatively, because they block the flow of *chi* so that it cannot move smoothly from the *Tan Tien* to the limbs. Too much muscle tissue also creates pressure on the internal organs, which is not beneficial. Muscles look strong, but they do not do much for your actual health.

Q: How can you prevent chi *from going away?*

Master Ni: Don't worry about it as long as you still have your productive body. Only worry about not making any negative application of *chi* in your life.

Q: How can you prevent energy from going into the wrong channels and going crazy?

Master Ni: This does not happen from doing *T'ai Chi*, but it can result from certain types of *Chi Kung (Chi Gong)* practice without correct guidance.

Q: What kind of Chi Gong *is that?*

Master Ni: It is the type of *Chi Kung (Chi Gong)* that is done by standing there and letting the *chi* move you. There might be a safety problem in that. If you read my book *Internal Alchemy* in its entirety, you will understand the purpose and correct use of such a practice.

    If you do not do enough *T'ai Chi* or *Chi Kung (Chi Gong)*, you will not produce any *chi*. If you overdo it, you will be worn out and will damage your *chi*. Do not make strange attempts or unprepared explorations of the mind.

    In all types of *T'ai Chi* Exercise, when you follow the teacher, your movement is almost like an external exercise that is not yet connected with your deep mind to stir your energy flow.

If you have a hereditary mental condition or if your nervous system has any hidden damage from your childhood and your *chi* is blocked, you may find yourself suddenly shaking, yelling or doing some other kind of uncontrolled behavior when you do *Chi Kung (Chi Gong)*. This is called, "The evil fire bursts out." You can prevent the situation by learning the kinds of *T'ai Chi* that we promote in this book.

If you do *Chi Kung (Chi Gong)* without correct guidance, you have to be careful. When you do Five Animal Automatic *Chi Kung (Chi Gong)* without the proper understanding or correct guidance, you should be cautious.

In general, there is nothing to worry about when doing *T'ai Chi* or *Chi Kung (Chi Gong)*. Some of you are interested in developing physical strength and more energy. Others may want to develop higher potentials on a psychic level, etc.

The Spiritual Meaning of Physical Movement

Master Ni's talk at the Chinese Community Center,
February 18, 1989

Whenever you do *T'ai Chi* movement or other internal arts with good concentration, you will be centering your life so that your energy naturally generates and grows. This is not easily seen, but when you practice day by day, your health and your physical and emotional condition will be greatly improved and longevity can be attained. Doing *T'ai Chi* movement helps generate *chi*. From the achievement of *chi*, you can go further to reach the subtle level of *shen* or spirit. This is accomplished in steps; it is too difficult to jump directly to the spiritual level and expect realistic benefits.

In general society, people take one of two attitudes about spiritual energy. If they have an intellectual attitude, they do not believe in it, because they have not experienced it. The other attitude is the more conventional one, characterized by people who are followers of something or someone else. They have not experienced their own spiritual energy, and they are just willing to believe what somebody else has said about it.

Argument is negative, useless and meaningless. As students of *chi*, we need practical, matter of fact, step-by-step scientific attitudes without fooling ourselves into believing someone's description or someone's negative attitude toward the existence of the high level of life energy.

The learning environment for modern people is different from that of ancient people. Ancient people learned from a teacher's words. They did not have any difficulty accepting the teachings, so their achievement was much faster. Today, because we are intellectually educated, we have a lot of trouble believing. The benefit of our intellectual education, however, is that we are more objective.

I recommend that you stay at the level of *chi* without going too high to the delicate spiritual level, the reason being that modern life with its noise, speed, and unnaturalness can conflict with your development. When your energy becomes so subtle, something that happens a thousand miles or a million light years away is experienced as if it happened in your back yard. You know everything. With that kind of sensitivity, how can you stand the noise of modern life? When an airplane shakes the air in the sky, you feel it intensely because you have become so delicate, subtle, and gentle. It feels like the plane has flown right into your lungs. When the spiritual size of your life being is much larger than your physical being, you are affected by everything around you.

On the one hand, I hope that modern people can develop spiritually so that they can rid themselves of negative cultural influences. On the other hand, how does a spiritually developed being cope with the turmoil of this modern, noisy, dusty, polluted world?

Doing something to increase your health is of utmost importance to your life. Most people do not need any special training or teacher to teach them anything higher than that. Although all people are equipped with three spheres of energy, a person who learns more but only has partial spiritual development will experience some difficulty. If you become more spiritual, more delicate, and more sensitive, then you will suffer as the modern world gets worse and worse.

The traditional books of the Way, or Tao, are mostly collected in the *Taoist Canon*, which takes a long time to study and read. Most of its contents are not highly useful. Only those who are already spiritually developed or who have had special instruction can see the true blue sky above the clouds and can tell which parts are truly helpful and which are not. The general public usually does not see any value in any of the teachings and therefore does not respect them. Even if an undeveloped person is interested in them and reads them or asks someone to translate them, they will still not understand the meaning because they lack the special training.

There is a gap between the spiritually developed minds of the ancients and the intellectually developed minds of modern people. Modern people do not believe or trust anything that they do not understand, so they destroy much of the great heritage from their lack of respect for high achievement and reality. However, after they learn about it, they come to realize that such things as *Chi Kung (Chi Gong)* are great proof of the advantage of the ancient culture and way of life.

The secret of spiritual achievement is that once your material sphere is strong enough to support your life, you should gather your mind, spirit, and physical energy to engage in the enterprise of a long, healthy life. The Way is open. It belongs to anyone. There is no secret in the teaching of the Way, but its profundity truly impresses people who think it is secret and mysterious.

Many teachers are selfish. Others do not teach true methods to general students. Either the teachers themselves are not highly achieved, or the student has not yet come to the right stage, and therefore the teacher has difficulty talking about it. Some teachers of *T'ai Chi chuan* promote the method they teach just for general health, because general health is more valuable than becoming a champion. The martial art that makes people champions is also the art that makes people short-lived, just like the modern iron machines that build muscles. It is not your muscles that live long, but your soul.

In learning the Way, we worship three types of purity which are called the Three *Ching* or *San Ching. Ching* means cleanliness and purity. When your body is pure and without any sickness, you have achieved the level of *Tai Ching.* When your mind is pure and untroubled, you have achieved the level of *Shang Ching.* When your spirit is pure and unconfused, you have achieved the level of *Yu Ching.* To achieve all three is our goal. That is the most truthful and useful trinity. The true student of the Way learns something for oneself and works on oneself, because the *San Ching*, the Three Purities, are contained within your own life being, not in some temple. Wooden statues can be spiritual symbols, but for successful spiritual development, the main enterprise is the work you do on yourself.

Chapter 7

The Breath of Life

In ancient times, the man of natural truth slept without dreams and was free from worry in his waking hours. He ate without interest in seasonings, and his breathing grew deeper and deeper. Such a pure, natural being breathes with his entire organism, not just superficially. Ordinary men breathe shallowly, in their throats; that is why, if they are arguing with someone and are defeated, the words catch in their throats. As their desires and ambitions grow, their organic wholesomeness becomes weakened.

- Chuang Tzu

Q: Would you talk about breathing?

Master Ni: This is a big subject, but I can make it small. If you live in a natural place, it is great to breathe fresh air. In a city that has smog, however, I would avoid breathing practices. I think mental practices for internal and external attunement would be more beneficial in this situation.

When you practice in the countryside with great natural support, there is less question of what to do and how you do it. When you live in a big city, your survival strength lies with the mind and spirit.

Q: What happens when we breathe during our chi *practice?*

Master Ni: The energy function of the body acts in opposition to the physical motion. Thus, when you stretch or make a big movement that opens the body up, exhale. When you contract and gather yourself back together, inhale so that the energy comes back to your center.

The natural motion of *chi* inside the body reverses the ascension and descension of the breath. When you inhale, your breath comes down; by internally pressing the air down, you create a pressure so that the energy rises. When you exhale, you naturally release air pressure from inside, and the energy sinks. This is how *chi* functions in opposition to physical movement.

Dr. Maoshing Ni: Breathing is an integral part of any kind of *chi* exercise such as *T'ai Chi* Movement, Eight Treasures and *Dao-In*, because breathing patterns allow you to create a rhythmic flow of *chi* in the body. Because the composition of *chi* within the human body is related to the intake of oxygen, the breath of life and the life force are intimately related. Mastery of the breath allows you to gain mastery over all the energies in your body.

Learning to breathe properly helps quiet the mind. Ideally, you should breathe long and deeply, slowly and rhythmically. One goal is to breathe so quietly that you cannot hear your breathing. The more refined the breath, the quieter it is.

Q: Are chi *and breath the same thing?*

Master Ni: In Chinese, *chi* is breath. When *chi* is associated with emotion, it is expressed as emotion. Thus, the word for "air" and for "internal emotional condition as *chi*" are the same, but they are understood differently according to the context. In English, breath is the air and *chi* is the internal energy.

Dr. Maoshing Ni: As my father says, *chi* and breath are different. *Chi* comes in many forms. For example, there is electrical energy, magnetic energy, and heat. Air, which is composed of many different elements, including oxygen, is a type of energy too. Air fuels the body and contributes to the composition or health of *chi* within the body, but the life force within the body is not merely air. The air we breathe is merely one part of our life being.

Q: How should we breathe when practicing chi *exercise?*

Dr. Maoshing Ni: In the beginning, breathe naturally. Eventually, try to breathe with your abdomen only. Breathing through the mouth is very shallow, so breathe through your nose. This encourages diaphragmatic breathing and allows you to pull the energy all the way to the abdomen, to the root.

Q: Is it necessary to do any kind of breathing practice, aside from what we do in chi gong *or* t'ai chi *exercise?*

Master Ni: I have given guidance for different practices on other occasions.

There are a great number of breathing practices for specific purposes. The breathing practice I recommend here is peaceful inhalation and exhalation, which harmonizes with each relaxed movement. Healthy breathing habits can be built by doing gentle movements that conduct *chi* throughout the body.

The principle for breathing is "deep," "quiet," "thin," "gentle," "slow," "controlling," and above all "naturally rhythmic." It is not suitable to focus on the breath rather than on the movement. Breathing is the go-between that confirms the marriage between the mind and body.

Q: Are specific breathing practices for advanced students only?

Master Ni: Breathing is important at all levels. An advanced student needs to look for an advanced instructor.

Pure internal energy practice does not emphasize muscles or special breathing techniques. The breath should have a natural rhythm, and the energy should move in synchronization with the breath. In this way, you expand yourself spiritually. After you have learned and practiced the movements for a number of years, you will go beyond the physical movement.

Dr. Maoshing Ni: My father has always taught us that breathing is something that everyone takes for granted, but the importance of breathing cannot be overemphasized. A person cannot live more than five minutes without breathing.

Have you ever noticed that when children breathe, their bellies naturally move in and out? That is because they breathe from their abdomens with natural diaphragmatic breathing.

When adults lose the habit of diaphragm breathing because of various anxieties and pressures, their breath begins to move up into the chest area. As one gets older, or if one is afflicted with illness such as asthma or other types of respiratory problems, the breath begins to move even higher. Most people on their death-bed, particularly terminally ill patients, breathe only as far as the throat. Suddenly, the breath escapes and the person passes on.

Thus, the principle of good breathing is to root the breath as low as possible, in the abdomen. Many scientific studies have been done on breath control and metabolism. If you control your breath, consciously slowing it down to a certain rhythm and using diaphragmatic breathing, you can actually slow down your metabolism and nervous system too. This induces a state of calmness and meditation.

For most people, diaphragmatic breathing feels unnatural, although it is the most natural way to breathe. To restore this kind of breathing may take some time. It definitely requires a conscious effort. An easy way to begin is to put your hand on your abdomen and inhale, inflating the abdomen. As you inhale, the hand should move forward as the abdomen expands. Then, as you exhale, the abdomen should contract and deflate. This is basic diaphragmatic breathing.

When you breathe deeply, many things happen on a physiological level. First you efficiently expel the carbon dioxide from your lungs and system. You also take in more oxygen, which is beneficial for the whole body on a physiological level. Second, when you breathe diaphragmatically, you gain more energy. Exercising the diaphragm muscle also exercises the visceral organs and increases the circulation in of blood in the abdomen. Increased circulation is beneficial, because it means that more waste products are transported out of the viscera and more nutrients and oxygen are brought back in to nourish the organ systems. Thus, with deep breathing, one will have increased vitality.

It is well known that good athletes have mastery over their breath. The art of rhythmic, deep breathing is the secret to having a competitive edge. Statistics also show that opera singers have a longer than average life expectancy. This has a lot to do with the fact that they breathe diaphragmatically, which maximizes their intake of air and the expulsion of the various toxic gasses from the body.

Mastery and control of the breath also impacts other functions of the body such as pain control, because the central nervous system responds to the breath. Usually when one is in a panic, the adrenal gland is stimulated. When the fight or flight response kicks in, one begins to hyperventilate. By learning to master one's breath, especially by breathing rhythmically and deeply into the abdomen, one can control that instinctive response.

We should also consider breathing patterns during sleep. When people sleep on their backs, their breath is shallow because the lungs are compressed. Sleeping in that position therefore causes a lack of oxygen to the brain, and people who sleep on their backs tend to wake up a little groggy. The ideal way to sleep is on your right side, in a fetal position, which allows the lungs room to move.

Q: If we live in an environment that has bad air, is there something we can do to minimize the effects of pollution? You've got to breathe, but should you breathe shallowly in such a circumstance?

Dr. Maoshing Ni: That is a good question. Get out of that place as soon as possible. You are directly affected by your environment, and if the place has bad air, it will eventually contribute to bad *chi* if you stay there long enough.

People get sick in buildings that are totally enclosed and where there is very little oxygen pumped in from the outside. The sick building syndrome contributes to many different kinds of illnesses and diseases, causes stress and ultimately leads to a loss of productivity. If you encounter such an environment, yes, breathe shallowly. This is where breath control becomes useful.

Let's say you are visiting a factory or are near a dry cleaner or industrial plant that emits toxic fumes. Inhaling toxic gas is dangerous, so you want to breathe shallowly and maybe hold your breath as long as possible until you can get to a place where you can breathe fresh air.

When you practice *Chi Kung (Chi Gong)* and other *chi* exercises, you want to practice in a place that has good supply of fresh air, such as a forest where there are a lot of plants. During the day, plants take in carbon dioxide and give off oxygen as a by-product. If you practice indoors, there must be good cross ventilation to have a fresh supply of air. It is also helpful to exercise near the ocean, because the ocean is a good source of fresh air.

On a comic note, one must beware not to inhale one's own or other people's flatulence because it is methane, which is actually a toxic gas.

Our atmosphere shields us from the harmful ultraviolet rays of the sun, or else we would be burned. It is commonly known that the use of certain gasses destroys the ozone. A lot of blame has been placed on hydrofluorocarbons emitted by air conditioning units, automobiles, etc., and also on carbon monoxide and various types of carbon gasses, but did you know that methane is the single largest contributor to destruction of the ozone layer? About 40% of the destruction comes from the 5 billion people and animals who sometimes create methane gas. It goes into the atmosphere and burns a hole in the ozone. By simply improving their digestive systems, therefore, everyone could help minimize the destruction of the environment.

Master Ni: I would like to conclude our discussion with a story. Once, when I was in Taiwan, I was traveling in the third class section of a crowded train. As I stood there, I saw a farmer with two bamboo containers that Chinese people use to carry their heavy belongings, balanced by a pole on their shoulder. They put their belongings in two cloth bags or jars of equal weight, one on each end of the pole, and then balance the pole on their shoulder. The farmer I saw had two jars filled with water on his pole, and rather than use his hand to hold the safety strap like everyone else on the train, he kept his hands in the containers, constantly stirring the water. I asked him, "Why are you doing that?" He replied, "There are some small fish that have just hatched. If I don't do this, they will die, because they need oxygen."

Just like those little fish, all life needs healthy stimulation, moving and breathing well all the time.

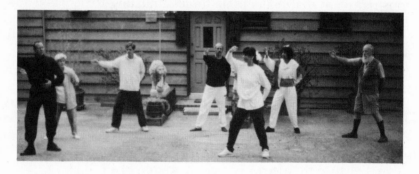

Chapter 8

Mind: The Sensitive Partner

When it comes to caring for their bodies and managing their minds, people are usually haphazard and careless. They stray from a natural life, depart from their inborn nature, destroy their form and spirit, and follow the crowd. - Chuang Tzu

The heart of Tao is the heart of peace.
It is not disturbed by the mind.
The heart is the mind that has no thought.
The mind is the heart after it falls into contemplative activity
and engages in busy thinking. - Chen Tuan

The great majority of us are required to live a life of constant, systematic duality. Your health is bound to be affected if, day after day, you say the opposite of what you feel, if you grovel before what you dislike and rejoice at what brings you nothing but misfortune. Our nervous system isn't just a fiction; it's part of our physical body, and our soul exists inside of us, just like our teeth are in our mouth. The soul cannot be forever violated with impunity.
- Boris Pasternak, *Doctor Zhivago*

Q: What about the mind? Should people do any kind of visualization when practicing chi *exercises?*

Master Ni: The mind is an important subject. When you exercise, your mind needs to concentrate on what you are doing or on specific instructions. In general, I think my book *Mysticism: Empowering the Spirit Within* can help to develop your mind.

Q: I really wonder about using the mind in chi *practice. Some people seem to focus more on visualizing the* chi *flow, etc., than on doing the movements. Others seem to think too much about what is in the next movement, etc. Concentration and thinking seem to be different.*

Master Ni: Concentration means that the mind is connected with the movement, not separated by its own thoughts.

Q: I have noticed that if I am thinking about something else when I exercise, I do not do as well.

121

Master Ni: Whatever exercise you choose to practice, concentration will increase your energy. It can also help you overcome your physical problems.

From an internal viewpoint, gentle movement leads to internal harmony. It is my personal experience that it is hard to practice when your mind is not calm and you are troubled. If you force yourself, you will damage yourself. Unity between the internal and external cannot be forced.

Q: Is there any special mental attitude that can help our chi exercise?

Master Ni: The best attitude is no attitude. Hold no preconceptions or preferences. If you experience bad things, immediately remove all thoughts of the bad experience, because each moment is new. Do not hold onto anything, good or bad.

Q: What should I think about when I practice T'ai Chi?

Dr. Maoshing Ni: Your mind should be passively active when you practice so you can be clear and precise about the message you are sending to your body. When your mind is garbled, like a computer with its memory in random places, you cannot be very clear in your commands, and your commands cannot be responded to with precision and speed. Thus, first you have to unclutter your mind so that you can focus. This is what it means to be passively active.

Visualization during *chi* exercise, such as visualizing a crane stretching and so forth during Crane Style *Chi Gong*, is all right.

Q: Quieting the mind is easy to say, but not so easy to do. I find that focusing on the movement helps. Would you say more about the commands of the mind? What does it mean for the mind to command the chi?

Master Ni: The mind affects the flow of *chi* by causing a disturbance. This is why you need to keep the mind inactive while you do movement.

Q: I'm not sure I understand. How do you use the mind to command the chi?

Master Ni: Usually each movement and each posture guides the energy to move in a certain direction. Without any interruption from your thoughts, that purpose will naturally be fulfilled. Gentle movements are slow, so it is easy for your mind to play hooky and escape to other things. The correct use of the mind is to join the body and the movement without going off on a tangent of wanton roaming. You cannot achieve this in one day, this is why it is called spiritual cultivation.

In the countryside of China, children raise snakes as pets by keeping them in a piece of bamboo. The snake always sticks its head out of the bamboo, and the children put it back in, again and again. The mind is like a snake, and the bamboo container is your body; they should always stay together. Do not let your snake stick its head out of the bamboo. There is a natural marriage between the mind and the body, but most people's habit is to let the mind wander away. They divorce all the time, because the mind has fun outside of its "house." If you understand this, you know that all movements are just ways to put the snake back in the bamboo.

Some *T'ai Chi* teachers are preprogrammed to say, "This is how you move. If anyone becomes aggressive, this is how you need to respond." If those thoughts are held in your mind, then your movements will be totally different than if you were to think, "This movement and practice is nurturing my energy and harmonizing my entire being."

Q: Is there a useful visualization for T'ai Chi practice? For example, visualizing moving like a crane, visualizing an opponent or opposing force, visualizing the flow of chi, visualizing a fire in the tan tien, etc.

Master Ni: There is no need for imagery. Just watch what you are doing and unite the mind with the body. The mind is not your thinking, but your awareness. Unification is the Integral Way.

Visualization is an internal exercise, and movement is an external exercise. Visualization can achieve the purpose on a subtle level, because the energy flow listens to the mind.

In some *Chi Kung (Chi Gong)* practices, particularly religious *Chi Kung (Chi Gong)*, there are different types of visualization that can be therapeutic for people who have a lot of illusions. If your mind is sick, that type of practice can be beneficial. However, pure concentration is better than complicated visualizations, although the purpose of both is the same.

In general, there is no moment when your mind is not active, whether you are awake or sleep. If the mind goes its own way, your "house" is left unattended or haunted by scattered memories. Spiritual cultivation can unify your three partners: body, mind and spirit.

Q: Does our mind really affect us very much?

Dr. Maoshing Ni: The mind can have a direct biochemical influence on a person's life. For example, when one visualizes a happy occasion, a pleasant thought or a beautiful place versus a frightening and unpleasant experience, situation or place, the body responds immediately in a corresponding way. Therefore, mental mastery allows an individual to begin to control one's body.

This is exciting, because it can be helpful for something as simple as having cold toes. If a person can turn their mind on and warm their toes up in 15 minutes, that is having direct control over one's body.

Modern science has been able to measure the activities of the brain with the ECG and EEG. Brain waves are *chi*. Each time you think or do not think, there is a different wave or transmission of *chi* or energy. Whatever is conceived in your mind will communicate inside and outside of your body.

Master Ni: In social situations many people can manage themselves externally, but internally they feel terrible. Many bad thoughts and emotions arise because they are stressed or have an internal problem, so they have trouble. When you do gentle physical movement, however, first you find internal peace. Then you find external peace, so you are at peace in both parts of your life.[8]

Q: How does chi *exercise affect the mind?*

---

[8]I would like to refer you to my book *The Key to Good Fortune is Spiritual Improvement* for information about how the mind affects your life.

Dr. Maoshing Ni: The practice of *chi* exercise can help prevent degeneration of the brain and diseases such as Alzheimer's. They still do not know what causes Alzheimer's disease, but some preventive steps include keeping the mind active and eating a low-fat diet. Since *chi* experiments are conducted on humans rather than animals, concrete conclusions are always slower.

Q: I read somewhere that there are different ways of thinking and of using the mind, and that the mind can be improved.

Master Ni: Some of my books discuss mental improvement in depth. In particular, the *Workbook for Spiritual Development* contains an entire chapter on improving the mind.

Q: How do you get the mind and body to work as one?

Master Ni: At a subtle level, you already described visualization. It can be as simple as pure concentration on specific *chakras*, spots or points, or a specific part of the body. If you are realistic, you will keep your mind moving with your body during all movements, including all life activity.

When I first arrived in the United States, I was often visited by an attorney who had become rich through real estate. He had a group of interesting friends, mostly from the movie business, some of whom were also my patients. Although this person had a great interest in spiritual matters, he had a stronger interest in using drugs to create the illusion of happiness. One day he did not come back from driving his car on the Santa Monica freeway.

I suggest that you always keep your mind on what you are doing. The gentle movements eventually teach you to nurture the marriage of mind and body. I do not think anyone can really afford a divorce. Nothing is more holy than this realization. It is the Way.

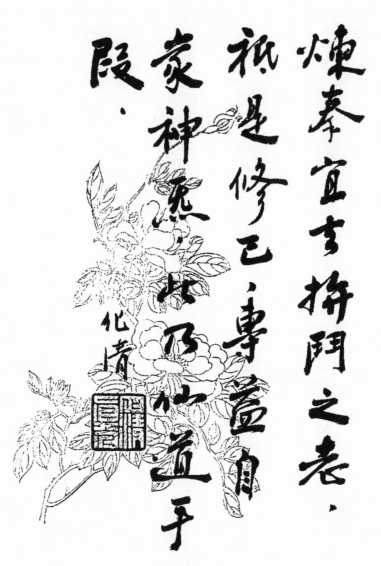

煉奉宜言搏鬥之志，
祇是修己專益自
家神氣，此乃仙道于
段。

化情

When practicing martial arts,
stop thinking about competing.
It is self-cultivation for the purpose
of self-strengthening.
This is the victory you enjoy
not for a short minute
but for a long time.

Chapter 9

Famous Practitioners of Physical Arts

This is what the people of the subtle path teach:
  if one has the ability to be a successful fighting rooster,
  one remains like a chicken and does not fight.
The wise one can be the deep ravine of the world:
  such a person lives with humility
  to maintain virtue.
Virtue is one's own harmonious spiritual energy.
The goal of the wise one is to return
  to the innocence of a baby.
Although the wise one is respected in public,
  the wise one would rather go unnoticed
  and live in privacy.   - Lao Tzu

Q: Would you please talk about some famous people who have practiced T'ai Chi *or other* chi *exercise?*

Master Ni: Lao Tzu, Chuang Tzu and many others practiced *chi* exercise. However, *t'ai chi* was the principle of their whole life, not just a form of exercise. *T'ai Chi* or *Chi Kung (Chi Gong)* movements were merely reflections of this deep principle of life.

For many years I have observed those who do movements like *T'ai Chi* Exercise or *Chi Kung (Chi Gong)* and those who do not do them. For those who do them, the minimum attainment is to look 5 to 10 years younger than those who do not. The median attainment is to look 10 to 20 years younger, and the maximum attainment is to look 30 to 40 years younger. It is possible to attain still higher. Each individual needs to adjust or attune oneself to make the best of such a profound practice.

Some other famous people who achieved physical longevity were the Yellow Emperor, Niao, Shun and Yu, all of whom lived over 100 years. Pong Tzu lived to be over 800 years old, and Lao Tzu lived 160 or 200 years according to Ssu Ma Chien, a reliable historian of the Han Dynasty. There was also Li Pa Ba and many others in the ancient tradition. A couple of Zahn (Zen or Chahn) Masters also enjoyed a lifetime of 120 years.

Today, many people worry not just about the length of their life, but about their ability to be healthy and happy when they are older. *Chi* exercise not only prolongs life, it improves your physical energy foundation for a more vigorous, healthy and happy life at any age. Self-cultivators appreciate the value of an enduring and untiring spirit that can live in a disturbing world.

I
Lao Tzu (571 B.C.E.) and Chuang Tzu (275 B.C.E.)

There are various styles or types of gentle movement that developed along with herbal medicine and acupuncture as part of a natural healing process. These movements were widely accepted during the Stone Age, but they did not become a spiritual practice until about 2,500 years ago, when Lao Tzu wrote the *Tao Teh Ching,* which teaches people to give up brutality and violence and become gentle, soft, harmonious and cooperative.

When Lao Tzu was young, he went to a teacher to learn the Way. In ancient times, there were no books or classes. A student learned from a teacher through observation and general conversations in daily life.

Lao Tzu learned an important lesson from his teacher Hueh Tzang. As a young man, Lao Tzu had difficulty accepting that the soft can win over the strong. One day the teacher asked Lao Tzu, "Which is stronger when they fight, my teeth or my tongue?"

To this Lao Tzu replied, "Your teeth, of course. They can bite many things, including the soft tongue."

Then the old teacher pointed to his toothless mouth, and said to Lao Tzu, "Look! Which one has survived, my teeth or my tongue?" Lao Tzu understood the illustration and later made it one of the main themes of his teaching. This is an important principle for anyone who practices self-cultivation through gentle movement.

This teaching was continued by Chuang Tzu, who wrote about an ambitious young man who spent lots of time and money on learning how to kill dragons. He was very proud of his achievement, but he could find no opportunities to apply the skill he learned.

Chuang Tzu was saying that people who believe their power is as strong as a dragon, as fierce as a tiger or as unbreakable as a boulder sooner or later run into trouble, because there is always someone or something stronger.

II
Master Kou Hong (283-363 C.E.)

Life can be learned through practicing the physical movement of the internal school. Master Kou Hong (283-363 C.E.), known as Pao Po Tzu during the Jing Dynasty (265-419 C.E.), was a model of literary and military achievement. He combined his knowledge of military arts with spiritual learning to attain a balanced personality and high spirituality.

III
Master Chen Tuan (ca. 885-989 C.E.)

All types of art have a background. Gentle Path T'ai Chi evolved from martial arts, but followed the philosophy of t'ai chi. T'ai chi philosophy was revived by the Sleeping Sage, Master Chen Tuan, who lived at the beginning of the Sung Dynasty. It was not until after his time that there was anything called T'ai Chi, although T'ai Chi movements originated much earlier and were reorganized again and again by different masters who all contributed toward producing a perfect form. The perfection of the entire form is its value, but it is rarely publicized in its entirety. The public can learn it on a simpler level than that of the masters.

IV
Master Tsan, San Fong

A clear record of the history of T'ai Chi Chuan was kept by Mr. Wahng, Chun-Shi, a great scholar who lived at the end of the Ming dynasty. His son Wahng, Pa-Chia wrote down Chen, Chow Tung's description of this art and passed it down to Chang, Shoong Chee and from him to Wahng, Cheng-Nang.

Much later than Kou Hong, Master Tsan, San Fong who lived during the Sung Dynasty (960-1279 C.E.) pursued the Way and achieved himself. He began to use the name "the internal school" to describe his type of martial art.

Later, another Master Tsan, San Fong lived during part of the Yuan Dynasty (1200-1367 C.E.) and the Ming Dynasty (1368-1643 C.E.). He further developed the art of the internal school. Because they have the same spirit, the internal school and the school of swordsmanship are actually the same school with different names. The internal school is the more popular of the two.

Many students thought that these two masters, both named Tsan, San Fong, were the same person because the names were the same. However, the first Master Tsan, San Fong was described as having started the art of the internal school by spiritual inspiration while carrying out his duty of protecting a delivery of herbs to the Emperor. While traveling to the capital, Master Tsan, San Fong and the carriers spent the night at a roadside temple. A spirit, the main god of the temple, Shaun Ti (the authority of the North Star), taught Master Tsan, San Fong the art of using the sword in a dream. The next day, he and his carriers were besieged by a group of bandits who wished to take the herbs. With a single sword, Master Tsan, San Fong defeated over a hundred bandits. In this way, without having learned external martial arts, he came to be respected as the initiating master of the internal school.

The later Master Tsan, San Fong is much more renowned for his immortal achievement, but there is no direct record of his being involved with the arts. Even so, it passed from teacher to students and he was believed to have started *T'ai Chi Chuan*. He may have further developed the art of the internal school begun by the former Master Tsan, San Fong.

It is possible that the two Masters Tsan, San Fong were actually only one person. It is also possible that they were two and the second continued the work of the former, but the truth is not known and is only a matter of speculation. It is not uncommon for a spiritual life to be like uncontrolled dragon energy. I accept what the teachers of the last generation taught without making any personal assertion.

Master Tsan, San Fong's history was recorded by the great scholar Wahng, Chun-Shi. His son, Wahng, Pa-Chia, learned the art from Master Wahng, Cheng-Nang, a teacher whom the father invited to teach his son. Wahng, Cheng-Nang had learned from Master Zang, Song-Chi. Master Zang, Song-Chi learned from Master Chen, Chow-Tung of Wenchow who learned from Master Wahng, Chung of Shensi Province. Wahng, Chung learned this art after several generations of direct passage from Master Tsan, San Fong.

The origin of the internal school was clearly given in the personal record of the son, Wahng, Pa-Chia. The principles of the internal school were also clearly given.[9] Wahng, Pa-Chia's writing was not intended for social promotion because it was a personal journal. He was a scholar. All other Chinese scholars at that time looked down upon any kind of physical art or work, including

---

[9]These principles were given by Master Ni in his book *Tao, the Subtle Law*. Some have been reprinted in this book, on pages 85-88.

martial arts, because they did not consider this type of learning as having educational value.

The question of whether *T'ai Chi Chuan* was the art of the first Master Tsan, San Fong has never been answered. There are minor differences in the names of the movements. The focus on single movement practice was emphasized more than the practice of the whole series of movements that we now have.

There is another anecdote about Master Tsan, San Fong. It was told that one day, he was meditating in Wu Tang San,[10] where he lived after accomplishing the special errand of carrying herbs to the emperor. There he saw a crane and a snake fighting and was inspired by them. The snake, by following the naturally smooth, winding and swift movements of its body, can usually escape the sharp beak of the crane. However, the crane has a long neck which is similar to the body of a snake. A crane can be trained, or learn from the snake, how to develop a similar movement; then the crane will not lose the battle. In other words, a crane needs to develop its skill. This confirms an important principle in physical art, which is practice.

Master Tsan, San Fong found this fight interesting and inspiring. He integrated what he learned from the snake and the crane into his practice and was believed to have developed the art of *Ba Gua* movement and further developed the art of the internal school.

Another account of the origin of *T'ai Chi* movement is that the first *T'ai Chi* movement was passed down from Master Tsan, San Fong to Wahn, Tzung, who passed it to two students. One student was Chen, Chow Tung of Wenchow, and the other person was Jiang Fa of Hunan. Jiang Fa's teaching seems to have disappeared.

The popular Chen family of Hunan, famous for *T'ai Chi Chuan*, declared that their *T'ai Chi* was developed by their own ancestors and that they had not learned from Jiang Fa. Although in reality their statement may be inaccurate, the descendants of the Chen family were truthful, because they were born much later and they could not verify what they thought they knew.

However, practitioners in a nearby town passed down a different story about the Chen family. They said that the Chen family of Hunan had learned from Jiang Fa and had spread the art of internal *T'ai Chi Chuan* to neighboring regions.

---

[10]San means mountain.

The many valuable skills and helpful knowledge that I teach were not necessarily the invention of my direct ancestors. However, they learned them, preserved them and passed them down to benefit other people. This is the principle of our family.

Q: Is there more that can be said about the practice of movement by Lao Tzu, Chuang Tzu, Kou Hong and Chen Tuan?

Master Ni: Lao Tzu did *Dao-In* and a sexual practice (a type of physical movement) that was disclosed by a scholar of the Han Dynasty, Liu Shan. Liu Shan interpreted Lao Tzu's philosophy as a sexual teaching.

Chuang Tzu practiced meditation and breathing.

Kou Hong was a great collector of spiritual practices. He did *Dao-In,* breathing and sexual practices called the Golden Medicine.

The foundation of my teaching comes from them and follows the same principles: to learn only the essence and to achieve yourself in a safe way. For example, in my own life, I speak and write as a service to people. When I do my practice of gentle movement, however, I am not pulled away by the world. I enjoy movement when I get up in the early morning, when I walk in the forest, and when I labor on the land. Thus you can see I also have some fun in my personal life.

Chapter 10

Doing Gentle Movement
Is Spiritual Learning

1

Doing the movement is spiritual learning.
It breaks down any meaningless vexations
  and impractical ambitions that you might have.
Inside, there are no more random thoughts.
Outside, there is no more attachment to anything.
You can only reach total fulfillment and self-nature
  by being easygoing.

2

Doing the movement nurtures your wisdom.
How can you live right without wisdom?
Vulgar wit is like fire and poison,
  it harms people and harms self.
You can enjoy being nice and cool
  with spiritual wisdom.
It looks ordinary and tasteless,
  but it serves your life marvelously!

3

Doing the movement is learning to be poised,
  whether you move or stay still.
Your mind is at peace.
Everything in the world continues to change,
  but your empty mind is powerful
  in transcending all evil.

4

Doing the movement is the best discipline.
No wanton desire, stealing or killing exists.
Neither do you find any joy in arguing.
You let go of all trouble.
Whether you experience gain or loss,
  you laugh.
The great victory is having subdued the self-satan!

5

Doing the movement is an offering to the Divine One.
There is no need to search for it.
The Divine One is everywhere.
In all places, the Divine One exists and is the same.
Do not bother to climb the holy mountain
        when you can find the trace of the highest God
        in your own heart.

6

Doing the movement is better than
        reading all the holy scriptures.
Without missing a day,
        you do the movement each morning and evening.
Even if you have read all the holy books,
        your perplexity of mind remains the same.
Worship the simple, original spiritual nature.
Find the freedom beyond all descriptions.

7

Doing the movement is better than reciting a mantra.
When you do it,
        the loving Goddess of Mercy is with you.
Your body, mouth and mind are cleansed.
All secret and sacred postures
        have the effect of repeating a secret mantra
        ten thousand times.
It is better to do one round of movement
        than ten thousand mantras.

8

Doing the movement is better than chanting.
No separation exists between the chant
        and your self-nature,
        yet chanting by mouth
        is not better than chanting by mind,

and chanting by mind is not better
than doing it with one's whole body.
Spiritual paradise is under your own two feet.
Bow to the Infinite Light.

9

Doing movement is spiritual learning.
Do not laugh at my craziness;
Physical movement contains all spiritual meaning.
The ultimate truth is at hand.
Spiritual learning does not create fear
    of life or death.
Many ageless immortals have set good examples.

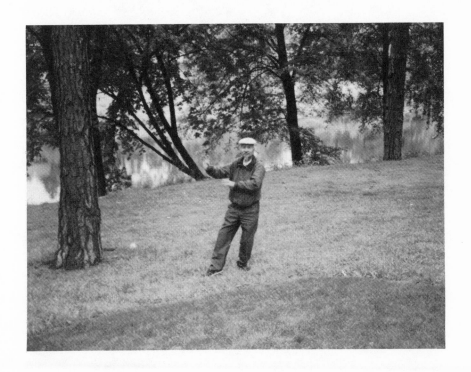

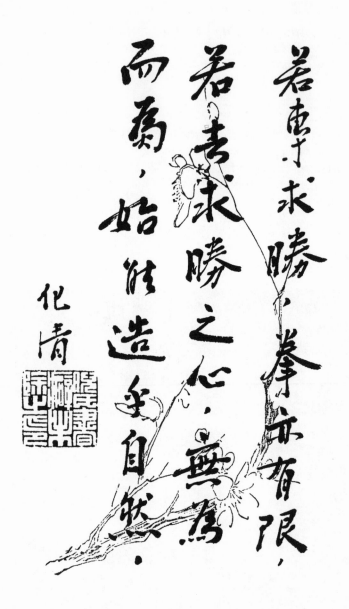

若專求勝，拳亦有限，
若去求勝之心，無為
而為，始能造乎自然。

化情

Fighting to win
    is very limited.
If you quit trying to fight and win,
    and enjoy practicing for nothing,
        then you attain the naturalness of the art.

Chapter 11

How the Physical Arts
Relate to Spirituality

The typical way of the world is to teach people
to get rid of weakness and become strong,
to remove softness and become tough.
However, the subtle truth teaches us
to stop using force and become soft,
to remove toughness and become gentle.

Those who are soft
can manage the strongest.
Subtle energy has no form,
thus it can go into and out of any space.
This is the great benefit
of being soft and subtle
and not using force.
Learning the subtle path
is not only something that you know,
but also something that you live.
Many people know that not applying force
brings greater benefit,
but few are willing to do it.
Living a life of no force
is the subtle truth of life. - Lao Tzu

T'ai Chi Movement is an Illustration of the Teaching of the Way
I

Q: Could you talk about T'ai Chi Exercise *and how it relates to spiritual development?*

Master Ni: *T'ai Chi Chuan* or *T'ai Chi* movement as an exercise is an important part of my teaching. Its movements illustrate important spiritual principles of everyday life.

We know that life is a matter of energy management. Whether your actions are wrong or right depends on how you project your energy. *T'ai Chi* movement can teach you how to achieve harmony by nurturing, managing, controlling and enriching your energy. It is a fundamental practice of the ancient developed ones, and of many modern developed ones, too. My *T'ai Chi* style is called the Style of Internal Harmony.

There are other special spiritual practices, but because *T'ai Chi* is tangible, it can be easily learned, and that is good.

There are two ways in which *T'ai Chi* movement helps a person's spiritual development. First of all, it can help you organize your own energy. When you are organized and clear, a potential confrontation can be transformed from a fight or argument, in which both people lose, to a situation in which both people gain success. Mutual winning occurs through harmonizing and yielding. By proper yielding, you may get more out of life than by fighting.

Second, you become more sensitive and thus do not allow any conflict or friction to occur in the first place. You are saved and other people are also saved. You can still achieve your goals, but without going to war with anyone. Thus, you benefit yourself and you benefit other people at the same time.

On other occasions, I have talked about the universe as an energy egg.[11] The energy egg, in previous generations, was interpreted as the *T'ai Chi* symbol, with smooth movement inside and outside, *yin* and *yang*, left and right, high and low, forward and backward, balance and symmetry, and so forth. It is the clearest illustration and application of the Way.

In our daily lives, we often find ourselves in hot or cold situations. How things turn out depends on how you manage them. If you do not learn *T'ai Chi* or the *t'ai chi* principle, you could become violent when provoked, not necessarily physically violent but emotionally violent by swearing or being stubborn or in your thoughts. Also, if you do not like something, and you fight it, you can make a small thing become bigger. If you fight to try to obtain what you want, all your relationships can become bad.

Whether it is a personal or business relationship, problems usually start from some small friction. Gentleness and sweetness are what you learn from *T'ai Chi* movement. Gentleness and sweetness are how you maintain good close personal relationships.

In our tradition, we do not teach you to surrender to the attacks of other people. We say that there is a way to live in the world and at the same time dissolve such attacks gently and tactfully. If you do this, people will not even notice that they have forgotten their reason for attacking. This is different from the religious teaching

---

[11]See *Power of Natural Healing.*

that tells you if your neighbor boxes your right ear, then give him your left ear also so he can do it to you again. How long can anyone sustain that? The practice of *T'ai Chi* teaches people to stay flexible when facing any situation.

After learning and practicing *T'ai Chi* movement, when you notice a potentially confrontive situation, you can move in a different circle to avoid it. Because of your gentle shift, your erstwhile opponent will be fighting only emptiness. If someone decides to hit you in a certain spot, by the time their hit reaches the spot, you have shifted to a new position and they have missed you. You not only protect yourself, but you also discourage the evil attacking force. In *T'ai Chi* practice, you learn how to make this type of gentle shift. In the spiritual application of the Way, you learn subtle movement to reduce external pressure.

In the world, we need to protect ourselves and others, but we do not need to become known as "a good fighter." Good self-defense does not mean fighting in all circumstances. So take advantage of *T'ai Chi* movement; the proper action does not come by fighting. I encourage you to make your best moves.

When people are young, they are sometimes inconsiderate, rough, aggressive, impulsive, irritable and provocative, because they do not yet know how to express themselves correctly. Anything square or thorny has sharp edges. Likewise, a person who is square or thorny cuts or wounds other people. Immature youths often have trouble because of poor communication skills. They seem to be cutting, and this hurts others. People cannot accept someone who is thorny or sharp. Hurting or fighting others not only shows a lack of maturity, it actually hurts ourselves.

In ancient spiritual terminology, there is a term that describes the opposite of provocative, impulsive behavior: "roundness." A person with "roundness" rolls smoothly along his or her way. The achievement of "roundness" indicates personal and spiritual maturity.

A young dog barks strong and loud. Truthfully, however, the louder a dog barks, the more frightened it is. When young animals are frightened, they usually react aggressively to cover up their fear. Making so much noise does not mean that the dog is well trained or experienced or that it will carry out its duty well. A well-trained dog does not bark out loud when it carries out its duty. Yet with training, animals can learn what is necessary. This illustrates the difference between being trained and untrained. Humans, of course, have much more potential than dogs or other animals. Through physical movement, people can achieve internal development.

If you learn this art, it will become a source of great joy in your life. Learning the Way is not boring. It is so much fun, because there are so many things to learn. It is like sitting and watching the ocean, the views and the energies are different each time.

II
Go Deeper than the Form

In the beginning, whether you choose *T'ai Chi* movement or *Chi Kung (Chi Gong)*, you must learn the external form, but the form does not necessarily stay the same for the rest of your life. As you progress, you move to another, higher level. The purpose of doing the exercise is not merely to be able to do the form. Ordinary people are always looking for external things to imitate and learn, and then they insist that a form needs to be done a certain way. However, the purpose of *T'ai Chi* movement is to attain something that is not formed. Nevertheless, you have to start with the form. Without a form, we would not have a way to teach you. For example, I teach the integral truth. The integral truth is not limited to verbal communication. Verbal communication can only convey intellectual achievement, but by means of certain forms, we can teach the integral truth by being it and doing it, thus enabling you to see and learn that which underlies the movements. My wish is that through movements that involve your personal activity, you will come to understand and appreciate the integral truth.

Often people ask me, "What is the Way?" I have attempted to answer this question at different times, but my words are an intellectual message. That is the nature of words. On the other hand, if people just see or follow me when I am doing *T'ai Chi* movement, even though they are not achieved themselves, they cannot help but notice that all the great principles of spiritual reality are being expressed and manifested. They may not know those principles intellectually, but they get a sense of them from watching the movement. People who go further and learn or master the movement themselves can have a direct experience of this.

Again, people often ask, "What is spiritual teaching?" It is the nature of the universe, and again I use *T'ai Chi* movement to answer them. In the moments when you practice gentle movement, you can find eternity in a flash. When you embrace all of nature, each moment, each movement and each inch of progression all hold the joy of timelessness and eternal youthfulness.

When I was young, I taught literature in a Catholic college. The priests were unhappy with me, because when people came to celebrate mass, which is a Catholic ritual, they saw me doing *T'ai Chi* outside. When they complained I told them, "Can't you see that I am praying too? You just do not understand my prayer."

"You should worship God in a godly way," they argued. "The Bible never said that God does *T'ai Chi Chuan*."

"If God does not move, there can be no universe," was what I told them. I define *T'ai Chi* as the best interpretation of Genesis.

III

The Flow of Tao, as Illustrated by *T'ai Chi* Movement

Tao, the Way, is the subtle law of all things. It is expressed through balance, rhythmic movement, naturalness, and the acceptance of differences. It can be the guideline for individual as well as social life, including economics and government.

The spiritual goal of individual self-cultivation is to follow the basics. When we discover that we are off balance or out of harmony, it is necessary to realign ourselves with the universal subtle law.

The subtle law is hard to describe. It is the principle of all positive and constructive virtues, yet at the same time, anything that is over done will produce a negative result. It is all good principles and it is no principle at all. Thus, the subtle law cannot be interpreted rigidly.

When you start teaching your children to talk, they do not understand what mama or papa means at first. You need to repeat it again and again for the message to get through. Highly achieved sages did not talk very often, because of the potential conflict involved in the relative sphere of language. I try to describe it well enough to help you begin to understand, that is all. When understanding comes, then blockage and the obstacles no longer exist. You know what you need to do, and you do it.

The sole purpose of cultivating oneself is to gather *chi*. To gather *chi* means to nurture your life and your vitality. Your life has different spheres. Life is energy. Anything that assists you in nurturing your vitality and your life can be considered cultivation of the Way. Life can extend to the subtle sphere too, so the cultivation of the Way includes the cultivation of the subtle essence and identification with the subtle truth. Basically, cultivating the Way means learning how to use simplicity to govern complexity internally and externally. There is a difference between diversity and unity. You cannot demand that everything be the same. For example, each leaf on a single tree is different, although they are all leaves and all belong to one tree.

The minds of some Westerners tend to make everything the same. I once lived close to a pineapple cannery where pineapples were cut into pieces and put into cans. Modern education also cuts people down to size and standardizes them until there is no individual differentiation, and their natural wholeness has been destroyed.

Each person has his or her own goodness. When a person finds that goodness, he or she will be happy in their life or their work. The problem is that people do not respect the fact that goodness expresses itself in different ways.

I used to do Chinese birth chart readings as a special service for some people who requested it, for a charge. I would mostly help a person learn what the goodness of his or her life is. Now, instead of giving individual readings, I am contemplating writing a book to unify Western astrology and Chinese astrology, if I am encouraged by a good schedule and an expert helper. The project is so huge, I really wonder whether or not I should put myself in that direction.

People look down on others because of social standards such as wealth, power and influence. I do not think that people can expect their children to follow those standards, especially when they have not achieved them themselves. If they truly knew the taste of money, power and influence, they would also know their pitfalls. However, because they have not achieved their own goals, they project their ambitions onto their children or other people. They do not let each person be natural and find their own goodness.

Who is to say what is good and what is bad? You cannot say that being married is good if a person is not happy, or that not being married is bad if a person is happy being single. People are different, and so are their achievements. Some can be leaders, and some can be associates. You cannot say that only leadership is good and being an associate is bad. The standards that society has set are unnatural.

Religions also set standards that they expect everyone to follow. These standards often have their source in psychological disappointment with life. Disappointment generally comes from expecting something or someone to be perfect, powerful and all-capable. In other words, the focus is on external standards instead of real achievement. That is the difference between following a religion and learning the Way.

To make real progress in life one must learn to break through personal obstacles. An obstacle is anything that keeps you from offering your most creative and positive service to the world. A breakthrough or spiritual awakening can only come after knowing the complications of worldly life. It takes a lot of work to break through a blockage and receive new light. Breaking away from external forces is a spiritual achievement. There is no limitation to how many breakthroughs each person can have. The responsibility is ours, and we cannot excuse ourselves.

When you see a performance of *T'ai Chi* movement, a calligraphy exhibit or a beautiful floral arrangement, you may conclude that they are simple, beautiful and gentle, full of symmetry and poise, analysis cuts things to pieces. It uses the mind to describe what you experience, and the description may be quite different from what you have seen or touched.

The Way can be described as an itemization of its virtues and beauty, but just like art, the Way is the unexpressed truth that was there before the description of it. For example, a master who does flower arrangements already has the beauty inside himself or herself and is looking for the material with which to express it. Once he or she has the right material, that beauty continues to develop and be accomplished.

I often describe *T'ai Chi* Movement as a way to express the integral truth. When you stand poised and ready to begin, the beauty and all the good principles are contained in your unmoved energy. Yet most people only understand the moved, arranged, and exhibited beauty and do not see the unexhibited beauty.

To worship the Way or Tao is not to worship the exhibited beauty of form; you can arrange forms in different ways. We worship the unexpressed, unexhibited beauty, truth and goodness that is unlimited. Once beauty is expressed, it is limited. However, the integral truth includes the form through which it is expressed as well as the practice. For example, if you wish to learn the Way through *T'ai Chi* movement, you will learn the *T'ai Chi* form. It is not the form that is important, it is what can be produced by using the form.

When you learn the Way and look for a breakthrough, if you do not learn the basics, how can you break through? For example, the Wright brothers developed the airplane from a bicycle. Should we, today with all of our breakthroughs in modern technology, start over again? Or do we start from the point people have already reached and look for further technological breakthroughs? This is why all existing practices need to be learned, achieved and examined; then you can achieve your own breakthrough. It does not matter what school you attend; what matters is your personal achievement.

Do not insist upon or become attached to the form of any practice. It is through consistent practice that your own excellence and breakthroughs come about. The form itself is not the breakthrough. Rather, through practice of the limited form, you achieve the inexpressible.

People who follow a religion tend to let themselves be guided wherever someone else leads them. They do not know how to further their own spiritual growth. It is true that religion can be utilized to achieve oneself spiritually, but unfortunately most believers become attached to the form of the religion and miss the essence. Most religious literature is written in a metaphoric form that describes something not easily put into words. For example, if you read Genesis correctly, you know that it is a metaphor. When you understand that the words are not literal, then your mind is not troubled by it, because you know what it means. Still, so many followers of Christianity believe that the literal words are the absolute truth. Since there are many different scriptures in the world, people argue and even go to war over which one is right. This is completely unnecessary and absurd.

Darwin's theory of evolution is also a metaphor. Do you wonder why Darwin's theory of evolution is not scientific? It is not scientific because no description is complete. Some descriptions are closer to the truth than others. Both Genesis and Darwin's theory of evolution express part of the truth, not the whole.

Beginning and intermediate students of spirituality often become religious and insist that what they practice is holy. A developed person does not always happily accept any form, limitation or ritual practice, because he or she is already beyond the rigid, practice of ritual and follows only the indefinable universal spiritual essence within himself or herself. All achieved masters in different traditions can be followers of the Way, although perhaps they would not call themselves that. Anyone who is still attached to a vocabulary, ritual or uniform, is still a student who is not yet achieved.

The highest learning of esoteric Buddhism is called the "Palm Print of Buddha." If you are really achieved, your palm must exactly fit the palm print of the great master. This is a metaphor for the coherence between his achievement and your own.

In Chinese Zen Buddhism, the highest teaching is called the "Seal" of Heart and Mind," which is passed from one master to the next. It too is a recognition of the same level of understanding and achievement. This is not a matter of rituals, customs, statues, temples or shaving your head but of spiritual reality.

It is from the formed that you learn the unformed truth. We do not worship *T'ai Chi* movement as a form; it is the thing behind the *T'ai Chi* practice that you wish to learn. I use *T'ai Chi* movement, esoteric Buddhism and Zen Buddhism as examples of transcending the limitations of form. The Way is the direct path by which you learn directly from your own body, mind and spirit, without needing to become involved in the indirect teachings of a religion before learning the truth of life.

A good teacher uses forms to teach the truth without particularly rejecting or emphasizing any form. But if I continue to do that, it will confuse people. If people come and ask me, "What about Christianity?" and I say, "Good," and they ask me, "What about Islam?" and I say, "Good," and they ask, "What about Buddhism?" and I say, "Good," then they would ask about all religions. If I always say good, then, what can they learn from me? They remain confused.

I have no disagreement with Christianity, Islam, Buddhism or any religion. I use the discussion of formed religion to teach the unformed truth of the Way. I would like all people to attain the Way by using whatever form they choose to reach it. This is my mission, and it is hard work for me.

Can you have sex and eat meat and be on the Way? Yes, as

long as the way you go about it is in harmony with the nature of your own being. The Way is not for people who think the Way is far away.

IV

Student Questions

Q: Master Ni, what is the Integral Way? How does it differ from other spiritual traditions?

Master Ni: Religions and most spiritual traditions are involved with the worship of a personalized concept of God. The Integral Way is not another mental concept, but the primary, essential energy of the universe, not merely the products fashioned from it. It is beyond personalization. It may take form, yet it may also remain formless. It is beyond definition. Using words limits its unlimitedness.

The Integral Way could also be considered as the school of universal knowledge and wisdom that has accumulated over thousands of years. This interpretation could be used to differentiate it from other traditions.

Tao or the Way is the essence of the universe that existed before the creation of Heaven, Earth, or anything else. It is the unmanifest potentiality from which all manifestations proceed. It is being, it is non-being, and yet it is neither of these. After things manifest mentally or physically, they are given names or titles. The names and titles are not the Way but are its descriptions.

This analysis can also be applied to the human mind. When the mind is perfectly still and has not yet formed ideas, concepts, images or attitudes, it is the pure, cosmic mind itself. This is so even if one is not aware of its existence. Actually, it is only when one is involved in something or is excited or disturbed that one is aware of one's mind.

Pure Mind in ancient terms is called "Poh." This may be translated as the Primary Essence. It is the fundamental power of mind. When pure mental energy connects with universal, unmanifest, creative energy, it is referred to as the Original Simplicity. In its unmanifest aspect the Original Simplicity is infinite and boundless. When it becomes manifest, it then becomes finite and limited.

The Integral Way is not a religion. You could say that it is a highly refined natural science. Religions were originally created in human society out of humankind's mental need to understand

and control the environment. They can take as many forms as the human mind itself can take. However, all theologies are merely creations of the mind and are thus secondary to the original cosmic Mind itself. The content of human religions rely on psychology and intellectual justification. Consequently, religion has little to do with the ultimate truth.

The Integral Way does not emphasize worship. Worship is a secondary, mental activity. When you move your mind by creating the sentiment of worship, you fashion something outside of the mind as the object of your worship. This traps your mind in the illusion of duality. Rather than invent an outside sovereign to act as his or her authority, the practitioner of the Way perceives the worshiper and the worshiped as one. When this person engages in worship, he is revering the objectification of his own true nature.

Relatively speaking, the goal of the Integral Way is the reunification of oneself with the primal, creative energy which is the essence of the universe. The highest, most refined energy within each of us is of the same frequency as the primal energy referred to as Tao.

Your life is one hand of the primal energy of the universe extending itself outward as your Self. It is not like a fish that has jumped out of the ocean. We are extensions of the universal power that has stretched itself outward, not only into humankind, but into all manifestations. Since we have lost our Original Simplicity or original essence through the habitual mental perception of duality and multiplicity, we need to restore it within ourselves. In Chinese, the Original Simplicity is called "*yuen chi*," or primal, creative energy. With *yuen chi* we can do anything. If we disperse or scatter the *yuen chi*, we can do nothing. Original Simplicity is not a doctrine, it is the substance of all beings.

A practitioner cultivates his energy in order to realize his true nature. The Way is not merely a matter of weekly worship. Self-cultivation is essentially the practice of various techniques for the purpose of refining one's energy to progressively higher and purer states so that one may ultimately reunite oneself with the highest realms of the universe. As an aspect of self-cultivation, the Integral Way also includes the practice of certain rituals or formulas in order to bring about a response from the divine, cosmic energy of the universe. These are some of the activities and non-activities that compose the Integral Way.

At the end of the Han Dynasty (between 140 and 185 C.E..), a Taoist religious movement came into being which vulgarized the original esoteric tradition of spiritual teachings. The Taoist tradition in China has, since that time, divided into two main groups and many even smaller branches. One group preserves the original spirit of Taoism as personal spiritual development, while the other is involved with superficial religious ceremonies. I belong to the former, maintaining the original spirit as natural potency. My tradition is not connected with the local religious customs of the various Chinese villages - so-called folk Taoism.

Q: In Chinese history, spiritual sages are said to have advised the leaders. Is it possible to influence our leaders to make a better world?

Master Ni: Occasionally, when the world is disturbed, achieved masters do come down to help society, but since China established the communist dynasty, spiritual sages have stayed in the mountains where political influence cannot reach them.

In a group of wild horses, the strongest horse or the one that runs the fastest becomes the leader. In human society, political leaders may be the best runners, but they never learn how to become good human beings. They only know how to kick and run like horses: "If anybody does not obey me, I'll kick you to death." Stalin and Mao Tse Tung both did that. When they were young, they had the same goal as everyone: to reform the world because it was unfair and unjust. However, once they were in power, they were not open to new ideas or new leadership, they just wanted to be in power forever.

Once I was giving a talk, and a young girl asked me, "Master Ni, since China is in trouble, why don't you go fix China instead of coming to fix me?" I told her and the group that every person has an individual destiny. Jesus could not refuse the cross. Mohammed could not refuse fighting. Lao Tzu could not refuse riding the buffalo out of China to go to the desert. It was my destiny to come to the West to make friends, because Westerners are now much more open.

The founding fathers of the United States established a government with a system of checks and balances to be sure that no part of government would overextend itself. That is democracy. You learn to respect others and others learn to respect you. This great political system did not come about suddenly; a long period of darkness in England and other countries preceded American life. Your ancestors suffered tyranny for a long time, but they found a new place to start over.

The greatest contribution of the American forefathers was bringing about a system in which there is no need to fight a war every four years to change leaders. People just spend some money, and there is a smooth shift of power. Politicians argue and call each other names on television, but the result is usually that the better horse is the winner. Each election, many people ask me who will be elected. You can easily observe who is the stronger horse. You do not need to guess.

In ancient times, people stayed in monasteries. Today, it is more important to be in contact with people and let them know that there is a different way of life. This way of life can make us better, lighter, happier and more complete. This way of life is different from just being attracted to external pursuits. We can avoid the destiny, suffering, and lack of growth of the majority. Personal growth and maturity are up to each individual. Nobody can truly help; it has to be each person's choice and action. Although China produces sages, the majority is still the majority. The horse is still a horse.

Let us do our *T'ai Chi* well, maintain our health well enough to withstand the pressures of living in the world, and not run to the mountains. Anyway, mountain land is too expensive to buy for weekend retreats only!

V
Conclusion

For generations people have practiced meditation, *Chi Kung (Chi Gong), Dao-In, T'ai Chi* and *Ba Gua* to achieve the same result as early students of "immortology." These practices are the foundational level of internal harmony. Spiritual attainment, however, is not something you can see or hear. Further discussion on how to achieve yourself spiritually can be found in my two books the *Esoteric Tao Teh Ching* and *Immortal Wisdom*. Your success in achieving the unseeable depends on what you do at the seeable level.

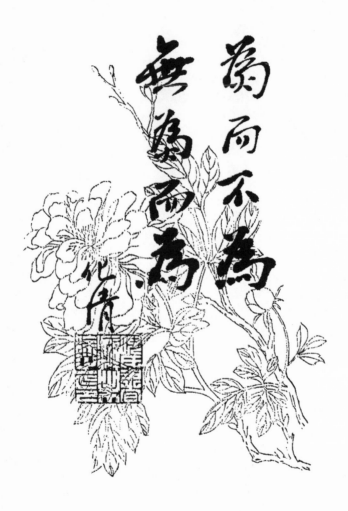

Do it for nothing.
For nothing, you do it!

Chapter 12

A Way to Find Spiritual Independence

Anything you can call a secret is not secret, because it can be told. The highest spiritual truth cannot be told. This is its secret. This great truth is by your side, also. - Hui Neng

Interview by Marvin Smalheizer
T'ai Chi Magazine, Wayfarer Publications
March 21, 1989, Malibu, California

Marvin: I would like to know some of your thoughts about the basic principles of Taoism and why the people of the United States are attracted to it. Is it for the right reasons or the wrong reasons? What are some of the problems that people encounter in understanding and practicing it?

Master Ni: It is my perception that Western minds direct their energy outward for the most part. This has brought about some improvement and achievement in life, such as scientific development, political democracy and free economic activity. These are the contributions of the Western world. I would say that Westerners manage better materially or outwardly, but their internal lives are a mess. This understanding is based on my personal contact with Western people.

Eastern people, through long generations of working hard to improve themselves internally, have not improved the material part of their lives that much. If East and West can meet, there would be nothing left out. I think this would be a good life.

I appreciate the intellectual achievement of the Western mind, but that achievement does not have to leave out moral improvement. When people are intellectually developed without having a good moral foundation, something is wrong. By moral development I do not mean conventional religious discipline. Religion, for the most part, is a crutch that was developed for furthering the growth of human society as a whole, but a person only needs a crutch until he learns to use his mind properly and stay out of trouble.

Often, when people come to learn from me, they think this tradition is another religion like Christianity, Buddhism or Islam, but it is totally different. What I teach does not numb people's minds so that they cannot see the true problems of their lives and the world.

151

Marvin: Do you mean emotionally?

Master Ni: Yes, religion is mostly an emotional or psychological approach. The tradition of Tao is totally different. It promotes spiritual sobriety, in contrast to people who become drunk on religion.

Marvin: Would you say that people come because they are seeking independence?

Master Ni: Yes. They are seeking independence instead of dependence. The Way provides that. As a student of Tao you learn internal sufficiency and richness, not the poverty of a spiritual beggar. Beggars look for someone who will bestow salvation on them or serve them the truth on a platter without any effort on their part.

Marvin: Can a person follow Taoism and still follow Christianity or Islam or whatever?

Master Ni: Certainly. Anyone can use Christianity or Islam as a foundation to understand the deeper teachings of Tao, but once a person insists that what he has learned is the absolute truth, he starts making trouble for others. This is what causes the world's religions to fight each other over their different beliefs and value systems. They have totally lost sight of their true nature by placing their trust in an external standard rather than the real standard of human nature.

Marvin: They miss the internal standard.

Master Ni: Yes.

Marvin: So Taoism offers internal sufficiency or independence.

Master Ni: If you learn the Tao, you attain internal sufficiency, richness and abundance. This is its purpose. In this way, you not only help yourself, but you can also help other people. By contrast, if you live in spiritual poverty, you have nothing of true value to offer others. Such people can only promote what someone else has said or their own imaginary concepts about life and the afterlife.

Marvin: When people come to Taoism, they do not know what to do. Many people do not have the discipline or the patience for meditation. What techniques, internally or externally, does Taoism promote?

Master Ni: At first, discipline is not usually required, because discipline is an achievement in itself. Once you see the value of certain practices, however, then you do them by yourself. For example, if you smoke, only when you understand its real harm will you finally give it up. It is a matter of personal growth.

We do not start by imposing discipline. We are new here, and there is no cultural background for the teaching of Tao. Actually, the same problem exists in modern China too. The real problem is the lack of understanding. So much religious conflict in the world is due to the lack of deep understanding of the truth.

Those who are interested in learning the Way need to attain some understanding first. Once you understand, then everything else will follow. If you do not understand, and only rely on a teacher to impose discipline on you, then even good discipline can be a poison, like unhealthy food that stays in your stomach undigested.

Marvin: So to make it a part of themselves, they have to see how to open their minds in their own lives?

Master Ni: The integral truth is a built-in system in each individual life. It is not an external thing, it is inherent in the individual. When people read my books, if the subtle capability for deep understanding is already there, the books are easy to understand, because there is no separation between what they are reading and themselves.

Marvin: Do they become dependent on the books?

Master Ni: No, the books become the description of their lives as their lives begin to change and improve from the learning. At the beginning, they need the books as a witness, as a proof, as a side mirror that helps them see and understand their own lives more clearly. Then they will slowly put themselves together.

Marvin: What kind of practice can they apply in their lives? What can you recommend to people that have problems with their relationships, work or health? How can they apply the ideas or principles of Taoism?

Master Ni: With regard to principles, we usually say, simplify your life. This is a big principle.

More specifically, when I travel to teach classes, people have different problems and ask me questions about them. Then I respond. When it is something that pertains to many people, it is always put into a book and published. People who read the books can use the indexes to gather information to improve their understanding.

Relationships, for example, are a concern for many people. Let's say there is a disagreement between two people. Who is wrong? You, your partner, or both of you? How can you fix the problem? Is the problem even fixable? If it is not fixable, do not be insistent. Stubbornness is the source of tragedy. If you would like to live a life of tragedy, that is a personal choice. If you would like to improve yourself, then find a different way. There is always enough light to see the problem.

Marvin: One of the ways that people consciously or unconsciously try to find the Tao is by doing T'ai Chi Chuan. *How does* T'ai Chi Chuan *tie into Tao? How can they use those principles?*

Master Ni: *T'ai Chi* Movement has many benefits. For example, if people spend a lot of time doing quiet sitting or meditation, they may have difficulty driving on the freeway. Meditation and worldly life are two entirely different levels of life. *T'ai Chi* Exercise is mid way between the two; you can still live a general, practical life. Practicing *T'ai Chi* Movement is also a good approach to internal and external harmonization. It changes your personal attitudes, mood and personal emotion.

For example, many diseases are caused by a disharmony between the organs or in the nervous system. If you practice *T'ai Chi* Movement, in time you learn how to harmonize yourself and eliminate internal conflict. Also, by improving yourself internally, your approach to the outer world will not be so impulsive or aggressive, which only provokes the environment to fight back.

Marvin: For my readers, T'ai Chi Chuan *is very important. How does* T'ai Chi *embody some of the Taoist principles?*

Master Ni: When a student learns the form of *T'ai Chi Chuan* from a teacher and only does that much, his or her achievement will be limited to that much. If he studies the *I Ching (The Book of Changes and the Unchanging Truth)*, the *Tao Teh Ching*, and all of my books, he or she can put that understanding into their *T'ai Chi* practice.

For example, if you go to school, you learn many things that are not necessarily useful in your life, except perhaps how to make money. Yet once you learn the Way or study the *I Ching* and *Tao Teh Ching* deeply enough, everything you have learned will express itself in your *T'ai Chi* practice. It is wonderful; the realization of truth, balance, symmetry, internal and external harmony, and neutrality can all be seen in your *T'ai Chi* practice.

Marvin: Do you recommend anyone who is interested in Taoism to learn T'ai Chi Chuan?

Master Ni: I would say that modern students should not be so insistent about their school being better than others. Some schools promote the martial arts, but martial arts are very limited. Each student should also learn the principles of movement from the *I Ching*, and the principle of balance between *yin* and *yang* from the *Tao Teh Ching*. Those books are the source of *T'ai Chi* Movement.

Marvin: How about Chi Gong? *It seems to be becoming more popular.*

Master Ni: *Chi Kung (Chi Gong)* means energy generating. *T'ai Chi Chuan* or *T'ai Chi Movement* is a form of *Chi Kung (Chi Gong)*. Although it is more advanced and more organized in all respects, if you were to dissect *T'ai Chi* piece by piece, you would have *Chi Kung (Chi Gong)*. When you move the clouds or do any movement by itself, it is called *Chi Kung (Chi Gong)*. It is actually nothing more than semantics.

Both of these arts originally developed from movement practices called *Dao-In*, which I translate as energy conducting. *Dao-In* is a set of simple movements that are combined with breathing exercises.

Later, because of external demands, these movements became more martial in nature. It is always easier to promote fighting skills than internal cultivation. Now that people have more understanding and development, they are coming back to the *Chi Kung (Chi Gong)* type of movement.

Marvin: Is Chi Gong useful in terms of both health and spirituality?

Master Ni: Yes, although it varies with the level of *Chi Kung (Chi Gong)* that is practiced.

Marvin: Some people who want to learn Taoism get involved in esoteric practices and hear that they are harmful. How can they know that they are practicing something that is safe? I am talking about people who try to manipulate the energy into certain channels and then have a problem. What is safe and what should they look out for?

Master Ni: The safe way to go about practicing is from external to internal. First learn *T'ai Chi*, then let the energy flow naturally. This is better than trying to manipulate it. Manipulation is unnatural. For example, the orbit circulation can happen naturally. Once you have the energy strongly in the Lower *Tan Tien*, if you force it upward, it will also be strong in your head and perhaps cause high blood pressure. This is why it is better to follow the principle of naturalness. When someone tries to become highly achieved overnight, they go against the principle of *t'ai chi*, which allows things to happen naturally and gently.

Marvin: Because everybody is individual and has a different level of talent, what sort of time should they try to look for in terms of progress or practice? People have no idea if it should be one week-end, or two weeks.

Master Ni: Generally speaking, modern people do not have time to learn *T'ai Chi* in the morning. They can learn in the evening, from a teacher, but personal practice is most beneficial in the early morning. Dawn is a very beneficial time, energy-wise. The amount of time it takes to make progress varies from person to person. It is a very individual thing. For some people it takes many years, while for others the amount of time is shorter.

Marvin: Is the early morning beneficial because of the yang energy?

Master Ni: Yes. All achieved teachers, whether they teach martial arts or personal health and longevity, get up early in the morning.

Because most people work so hard in the daytime and sleep so late, I suggest that they not overdo it. I believe that twenty minutes will be good enough.

When you do *T'ai Chi* Exercise, do not do it too fast or too slow. *T'ai Chi* Movement itself is energy conducting. Maybe you are sleepy in the morning. If you do it too fast, you will have too much energy all day. It is like, when you drink a glass of water, you control its temperature so that it is neither too hot nor too cold. You are the one doing the *T'ai Chi* practice, so how fast and how long you do it depends entirely on what is most beneficial for you. You can always adjust it. Each day is different. Generally, around fifteen or twenty minutes is good enough. In the afternoon, around 4:00 or 5:00, if you do it once more for twenty minutes before the evening meal, that is good enough.

Marvin: How about people who do a standing exercise or some variation of it?

Master Ni: That can give you more *chi*, more energy for martial arts and meditation. I think because modern people do all kinds of things to damage and abuse themselves, they can learn a good art and it will not cause them any trouble.

Marvin: So you feel that is good, too.

Master Ni: Yes, when some people who excel in *T'ai Chi Chuan* stand there, no one can move them. It takes a long time to learn that. Western people use weight lifting to increase their strength, but achieved persons can increase their internal power by just standing. It is a different approach. I think what you do depends on your purpose. If you have more time and are young, you can do the standing meditation. Ordinary people find it difficult to control their emotions and their sex drive, but they need to release those internal pressures in ways that are truly helpful to their lives.

Marvin: Is there a different approach to the practice of T'ai Chi or Taoism at different ages?

Master Ni: There is always a common factor, whatever a person's age, but there are also some differences. Discuss this with a really achieved teacher; they will know what is good for you. If you study with a teacher who only promotes one thing, you will never learn the truth of what is good for you.

Marvin: Would you say that younger people face different problems than older people or that they have different goals in their practice?

Master Ni: I think that middle-aged people have problems too. Everyone needs to learn differently. For example, some people are more physical, and some are more intellectual. Few young people suffer from physical stress, so they can set their main goal to be the attainment of wisdom.

Marvin: What impact do you feel that Taoism will have in this country or the West in general? You said something about this in the beginning. How is it going to benefit Western people?

Master Ni: People do not realize that they create most of their own problems. Once they learn the truth of spiritual reality, they also learn how to correct problems so that they can live a better life. No one can really take your problems away from you; they can only provide a temporary solution. This is why you have to solve things for yourself, and why the learning of Tao is so valuable. The world's problems are similar; all problems are the result of spiritual undevelopment.

Many of the people who read my books for the purpose of increasing their understanding get together with their friends and form study groups. Through sharing and discussing what they read, they can learn how to apply the principles to their lives. We learn *T'ai Chi* Exercise and the principles behind it as a way to improve ourselves and our lives. Learning Tao or spiritual achievement is not just a matter of exercise, however, although exercise is one part of it.

Marvin: In what regard do people create their own problems?

Master Ni: In the United States, we now have an enormous deficit, because we have spent so much on national defense for 30 years. It is true that we not only need to guard our own nation, but other nations as well, because of the conflict between two different political systems in the world. Spiritually developed people would say that we need to find a good way to live without fighting about it, but in order for that to happen, people first need to develop their understanding of life and themselves.

Marvin: People talk about spiritual goals, and everybody has their own. Based on Taoism, what are some spiritual goals that people might be aware of?

Master Ni: There are two different levels of goals. Outwardly, I think we should work toward a just and reasonable society. Internally, there are several levels. One is the maintenance of health and normalcy in life, because life itself is natural. We are all children of nature. If you do not do anything against your nature, I think you will accomplish your life without regret. At another level, all life is one life. Is there something else beyond the cycle of reincarnation? The answer is yes, but that is a spiritual science that only the student of the highest spiritual ambition chooses to pursue.

Marvin: In Taoism, the high science is longevity.

Master Ni: You must remember, longevity is still limited to physical existence. One level of personal achievement is to live harmoniously with other people. Another is a special practice to achieve survival after your physical death.

Marvin: What kind of survival is there after physical death?

Master Ni: There is spiritual immortality. Because you were born into a different cultural background, you were taught that God comes first, then the world, but development actually progresses in different stages from low to high and from coarse to delicate. Human life, which is the combination of spiritual and physical energy, is an illustration of this natural process. When we talk about Heaven, we usually mean the spiritual energy of the universe or nature. When we talk about Earth, we usually mean physical energy. Human life integrates both worlds. From this foundation, you can achieve a truly godly life.

For example, some people have a good mind. A better mind is related to a better spirit, but the spiritual level is still higher than the mind. Usually the mind does not know that there is spirit. It does not know because there is a lack of communication.

Let us talk about a truly integral person. Ordinary people can separate themselves from the world, society or their family, but can they separate themselves from their own mind and spirit? They cannot, because they do not understand how to communicate with the internal spiritual authorities of their own organs. For example, sometimes we make a mistake, and some part of our body already knows it, but the mind is oblivious to objective reality. You see, the mind is the true student. It needs to experience difficulty and learn from its mistakes. Spiritually, you do not need to experience mistakes; you already know. This is why it is important to look for unity and communication between the spirit and the mind.

Marvin: When you talk about spirit, are you talking about something inside the body?

Master Ni: Yes, the spirit is actually a group of energies inside your body. You could call it your spiritual energy. To discuss physics without talking about the spiritual energy of a person does not present the reality of human life.

Marvin: After life, is there a realm where spiritual energy stays?

Master Ni: It is different from a world like this. There are "worlds" where different levels of spiritual energy and beings abide. People usually call them heavens or just Heaven. In its broadest sense, life is the process of continual birth and death. In each moment part of us dies and part of us is born. We like to have everything so defined, which can be done at some levels, but at other levels it cannot. Each of us is in the process of evolution. The whole universe never stops evolving.

The teaching of Tao promotes spiritual awakening, not drunken religious belief. Once you are spiritually awakened and no longer asleep, you can manage your life much better at all levels: psychological, emotional, physical, spiritual, etc. All moral problems are spiritual problems.

Marvin: Can you give us an example of some people here in the West who had some spiritual awakening that helped them with their life or in their growth?

Master Ni: I receive many letters from people who say that they have changed. In the beginning, because I did not give any external discipline, they depended on themselves to understand what life was about and how to improve themselves. It takes time to make progress, it is not like modern medication that works quickly to cure a problem. But it works; it really works. If I had come over here fifty years ago, I do not know that I would have found any friends. Now I have many friends and students who really enjoy this opportunity for development. They are not looking for some one to organize their lives for them.

Marvin: What is the reason that you do not give external discipline?

Master Ni: I only suggest a good way so that when they understand, they follow it by their own choice. It is not actually a discipline, but something for their own protection.

Marvin: What can people do to spiritualize their lives?

Master Ni: I think it is a matter of understanding. Spiritual life is so light. Once you totally spiritualize yourself, you do not need to rely on your physical form at all. That is what we call immortality, but that takes too long to accomplish for ordinary people. I usually avoid talking about it. To most people I say, "Live well, be happy, do not create any conflict with other people, and maintain a moral standard in all of your activities."

Marvin: Would you say that there are any central issues in Taoism that are more prominent today than in the past? What might be the key problems or issues of Taoism?

Master Ni: In China, the ancient achieved ones played children's games with undeveloped people, which resulted in the development of religious Taoism. The Zen tradition used Buddhism to teach undeveloped people. Today we need to move beyond the established practice of teaching people a religion before teaching them the truth. It is wasteful and confusing. By learning directly from life itself — our own mind, our own body and our own spirit — not only can we save time and energy, but we can also learn the plain truth.

In ancient times, each line of my books would have been considered an esoteric, secret teaching. Today I can openly offer it to the world. I do not mind who learns it; a good student or a bad student, a student who needs a long time to understand it or not. I do not mind. I just give it. In ancient times, it was hard to get one meaningful word out of a teacher.

Marvin: You mentioned that it is important to simplify life; it is hard to simplify Taoism, but sometimes it helps people understand. Are there certain principles that would give a sense of what Taoism is about?

Master Ni: The simplest book that teaches the Way is still the *Tao Teh Ching*. All other books about Taoism are just explanations of the *Tao Teh Ching*.

If I had to pick something, I would say one of the most important principles in spiritual learning is to simplify your life, relationships, emotion, diet and all things. Too many contacts and activities confuse people. One minute they read this book, the next they turn on the television, and all their learning is washed away.

There are a number of good suggestions in different books. I would like those who learn *T'ai Chi Chuan* to use it well: not only to do it, but also to learn the great principles of balance, poise, symmetry, harmony and naturalness. Those are also the great principles of the Integral Way.

So at the same time that people do *T'ai Chi*, I suggest they also read my books. The practice and the books work together for further development. If a student has a specific spiritual goal, then maybe in the future they can attend one of my seminars, but the basic principles are essential to all further development.

(Mr. Smalheizer's article entitled "Taoism: A Way to Find Spiritual Independence" was published in the June, 1989 issue of T'ai Chi Magazine.)

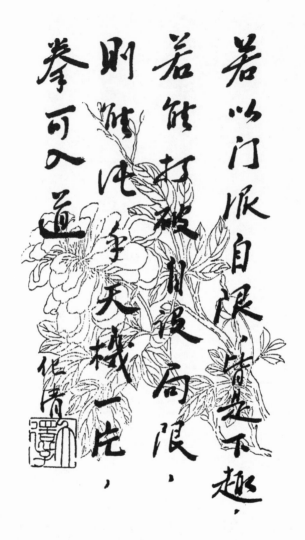

若以門派自限，皆是下趣，
若能打破門派局限，
則能池塞天棧一片，
拳可入道

There are lots of schools
  of martial arts and t'ai chi chuan.
If you insist upon dividing them into popular or deep,
  you limit your growth.
There is no higher school than being natural
  because that is where you attain Tao.

Chapter 13

Read to Improve Your Practice

In governing one's life,
    the mind finds support from the body.
Thus, the mind cannot be overly assertive
    in its own one-sided interest.
When a balanced life is attained,
    the unity of one's spirits is found. - Lao Tzu

Q: Is it important to read books to become good at T'ai Chi *exercise?*

Master Ni: Deeper understanding can be achieved by selective
reading. When you read the *Tao Teh Ching* and the *I Ching*, your
understanding will grow and you will know how to correct your
movements. It is not usually a matter of form, but of principle.

You might take half a year to read one book like the *Tao Teh
Ching*, but after that half year, your movement will be different
and better. If you continue to read good spiritual books, you can
eventually express everything you learn from them in your *T'ai
Chi* practice. It all depends upon how you go into it.

If you learn *T'ai Chi*, you should confirm your practice with the
principles taught in the *Tao Teh Ching*. If you have not yet read
the *Tao Teh Ching*, please read it. It will help you do *T'ai Chi*
correctly because of its emphasis on softness over strength. It dis-
courages people from looking for fights, although you can still
apply your training in an emergency for self-defense.

You need to have a spiritual goal when you do *T'ai Chi*. If you
do well in practicing *T'ai Chi*, you can attain the subtle truth and
know that it exists by your own development.

I

The Ancient Spiritual Classics Will Assist Your Learning

The *Tao Teh Ching* came not only from Lao Tzu's understanding
of universal law, but also from his long study of the *Book of Changes*.
Ancient versions of the *Book of Changes* were different from the
one we have today. Two versions, with different explanations of
the hexagrams, were used for many generations before the version we have today. Despite their external differences, the
fundamental principle of change or movement has not changed.

In the two ancient versions, the order of the hexagrams was
slightly different from the modern order. The version of the *I Ching*

that is now in use dates from the beginning of the Chou Dynasty, (1122-256 B.C.E.) and has been in use for over 3,200 years.

How was this teaching passed down from so long ago? It was simple: a set of symbols were developed and physical movement was used to teach the spiritual meaning contained in the hexagrams *Chyan* and *K'un*. Just like written symbols, gentle movement like *T'ai Chi* or *Chi Kung (Chi Gong)* is a natural way to demonstrate the truth of life. Movement is easy to understand and perform without intellectual training.

You can achieve yourself in everyday life by simply accomplishing what needs to be done physically, mentally and spiritually. Spiritual achievement does not come from sitting around waiting for the future to bring you a reward. People establish and follow religions without ever establishing a natural life. No religion can establish natural life. People can only live it.

II
Internal Spiritual Reality

The teaching of the Way is contained in the writings of Lao Tzu and Chuang Tzu, both of whom were great elucidators of the simple essence of nature and of the universe.

Spiritual knowledge goes back to the most ancient times when no written language existed. Spiritual experiences, knowledge of spiritual reality, and special methods for spiritual self-development were passed down orally from teacher to student. Some of these were written down in the late Han Dynasty (206 B.C.E.- 219 C.E.), and some were written down still later. The most valuable record of these practices is a collection known as the *Taoist Canon*, which contains instructions such as the "Script of the Great Cave." The word "cave" refers to the internal aspects of an individual life. "Script of the Yellow Court" is a simplified version of the "Script of the Great Cave." Many other important books are also different presentations of this same truth of internal spiritual reality.

Originally, the Chinese word *sen* was used to describe the internal truth of life. The English equivalent would be the word spirit or spirits. For example, people extract the spirit from grapes, rice and other crops to make wine. In this connotation of the word, spirit means essence. That was the ancient, straight way of teaching. After the advent of organized religions, spirit and spirits became God and gods, and the plain truth was kept secret from the general public.

Although there are many different religions, all religions are derived from the same natural phenomena of the universe: the sun, moon, planets and stars, light and dark, wet and dry, warm and cold, etc. Internally, the same spiritual reality exists in an individual that is in the sky. However, ideological stubbornness keeps people from seeing this truth and leads them into trouble. If spiritual teachers and religious leaders would teach the plain and simple truth to people, there would be a lot less trouble in the world.

It is important for people to understand the need to gather their own life energy and work to improve their natural spiritual condition. If they do not work toward spiritual self-development as their goal, they will lose touch with their own spirit and the great universal spiritual reality.

Q: What is the I Ching?

Master Ni: The study of the *I Ching* has reaped an abundant harvest of knowledge throughout its long history, which dates back over 5000 years. It is the foundation of Traditional Chinese Medicine, geomancy (the energy arrangements and relationship of one's environment, also called *feng shui*), military philosophy and strategy, Chinese architecture, and it is also the foundation upon which ancient spiritual understanding was developed.

Originally, the *Book of Changes* contained no written words at all. It only had signs made up of three or six lines, either broken representing *yin* energy, or unbroken representing *yang* energy. At first, the signs were composed of three lines. All of the possible combinations of three *yin* and/or *yang* lines resulted in eight main signs known as the *ba gua*. As time passed, later sages doubled the signs, making six lines, with sixty-four possible combinations. These signs are a concrete indication of all the energy manifestations of the universe, how they are formed and how they function.

Q: Could these combinations be expanded, or are 64 combinations the limit?

Master Ni: A group of scholars in Taiwan wished to develop the hexagrams to have nine lines instead of six and asked for my comment. I told them it could surely be developed further, but that is not the direction we pursue, because the Way is to use simplicity to govern complexity. The 64 hexagrams can be simplified to eight hexagrams. Those eight hexagrams can be simplified to eight trigrams, which can be simplified to *yin* and *yang*. With a simple principle, you can govern the entire universe.

A different way of dividing the sixty-four hexagrams into eight groups is by the five elements. The five elements are also divided into eight groups, but that is used for a specific definition.

The foundation of the *I Ching* is the cycle of *yin* and *yang*. Ancient "cosmic scientists" discovered that there is essentially one primal cosmic energy. In the stillness of the unmanifest aspect of the universe, the primal cosmic energy expresses a state of oneness. As it extends itself in the process of creation, its movement causes a polarization that gives birth to duality. The polar aspects thus created were designated as *yin* and *yang*. *Yin* and *yang* have many translations, such as positive and negative, expansion and contraction, construction and destruction, masculine and feminine, but they are not two separate energies or activities. The activity of one is inherently contained within and created by the other. For example, a symphony is composed not only of musical sounds; the silence between the sounds are also an intrinsic aspect of the composition.

The *I Ching* shows that the universe is one whole, but with two wings, like a man with two legs. In order to function effectively, the two legs do not fight each other, but work to help each other. For example, in movement, when you produce one kind of force to push yourself up and forward, at the same time you also produce a rejecting force. In Western physics, you say that for each action there is an equal and opposite reaction. This principle can be applied to everything, with *yin* and *yang* united as a *t'ai chi*. The *t'ai chi* then evolves into three levels of existence: physical existence, spiritual existence, and the combination of the two, which is mental existence. Human beings are one manifestation of mental existence and are a good example of the unification of the physical and the spiritual.

Through studying the *I Ching* one may come to know and experience the mysterious origin of the universe, achieve spiritual development, and keep pace with universal evolution. The *I Ching* is not a fortune-telling device, but an aid for the study and development of your own wisdom.

III
Cosmic Tour and the *Book of Changes*

Cosmic Tour is based on the principles of the *I Ching* in which the eight natural manifestations form an octahedron, a diagram with eight sides. This particular symbol is not of ordinary design. I would like to tell you how it came into existence.

Fu Shi, who was the originator of the *I Ching,* was inspired by nature. He divided natural phenomena into eight manifestations: Heaven, Earth, Fire, Water, Rain or Lake, Thunder, Mountain, and Wind or Wood. In earlier times, people experienced natural power through the manifestations of natural forces and called these forces the God of Thunder, God or Goddess of Rain, God of Mountain, Goddess of Earth, Goddess of Wind and so forth.

Fu Shi was more intellectually developed than the people who deified the forces of nature. He realized that all natural phenomena originated from one source and he devised a system to describe this natural reality in symbols. This arrangement, called the *ba gua* or octahedron, consists of eight hexagrams representing the eight forces.

The Rotating Octahedron and the Nine Houses

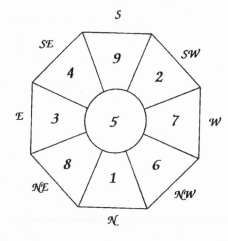

1. *The whirlpool*
2. *The rotating earth*
3. *The rumbling thunder*
4. *The gentle whirlwind*
5. *O*
6. *The changing sky*
7. *The effervescent lake*
8. *The majestic mountain*
9. *The transforming fire*

Cosmic Tour Movement has eight main sections that flow around a circle. Each section has eight small changes or transformations.

The movement goes from big transformation to small transformation. Eight times eight becomes sixty-four, just like the number of hexagrams in the *I Ching*.

Master Chen Tuan of the Sung Dynasty gave a numerical order to the eight main hexagrams:

> 1) Heaven, *Chyan*
> 2) Rain, *Tui*
> 3) Fire, *Li*
> 4) Thunder, *Chen*
> 5) Wind, *Sun*
> 6) big Water, *K'an*
> 7) Mountain, *Ken*
> 8) Earth, *K'un*

Each section is unified by this order.

A different way of dividing the sixty-four hexagrams into eight groups is by the five elements. The five elements are also divided into eight groups, but that is utilized for a specific definition. It has no relationship with this movement, so I just mention this for your information without going into detail here.

In the West, time and space are conceptually separate, as exemplified in the philosophy of Kant, but beginning with Einstein, time and space have not been considered separate. In the eight categories of the *Ba Gua*, the concept of time and space are unified. Movement through space creates variations of time.

Practicing Cosmic Tour brings enduring strength to your life, at the same time it teaches you the meaning of the hexagrams in the *I Ching*. It is useful and interesting for someone who wishes to do more than just read. It is something you can enjoy with your whole being.

Chapter 14

Special Topics

In governing one's life
  one learns not to be aggressive.
If force is used,
  internal harmony is disturbed
  and self-destruction will follow.
It is not often worth it to fight over material gain.
The gentle way can always help you achieve your correct goal.
                                        - Lao Tzu

Section 1: Swordsmanship is Not Only Done With a Sword

Spiritual Swordsmanship and the Internal School

The school of spiritual swordsmanship has a long historical background. It began with the tradition of the Way and combined martial arts with spiritual practice. All students were trained this way to different degrees. They deepened the art and kept their purpose strictly secret. They worked to achieve one goal: to deter and thwart evil. Some government officials were powerful and malevolent. Such tyrants would receive an ultimatum from the spiritual swordsmen to improve their harmful behavior or be punished. This was done by Mo Tzu's descendants or spiritual heirs. Their way of fighting evil was similar to western chivalry and the tradition of the knight errant.

By the way, the word "school," as it was used in ancient times, refers to a group of people who share similar beliefs or a common goal. A school was not a formal classroom situation like today's schools.

A spiritually achieved person in the School of Internal Swordsmanship could use his achieved mind to decapitate an officer who was a hundred or a thousand miles away. That kind of power is described in Chinese literature, but such a thing cannot be proven.

In the beginning, chivalrous swordsmen came from Mo Tzu's school. Later, the School of Spiritual Swordsmanship of Master Lu, Tung Ping and Master Tsan, San Fong followed the moral discipline of Mo Tzu and developed further to include physical movement, which could be converted into martial arts.

Now we follow all true sages who teach courage and who help the world through spiritual development. However, some people who learn spiritual development have a different understanding of worldly problems. No one should adopt the practice of killing anyone out of righteousness. The existence of evil in politics is due to two things: first, systems of monarchy and dictatorship, and second, the lack of individual development. The solution to bad government lies in education, not killing. The solution to the lack of personal development is obviously spiritual cultivation. Good self-government is the best foundation for social government. Thus, the focus of the spiritual practice of swordsmanship has changed to include teaching people how to be spiritual knight errants instead of social radicals who take extreme action.

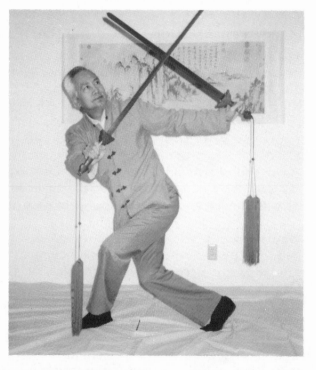

Transforming your own evil, not killing other people, is the only thing that can transform the world. In the first place, it is neither our responsibility nor our privilege to judge others. The enjoyment of killing is a symptom of spiritual undevelopment. Thus, if you wish to help the world, do it through developing yourself first and then through spiritual teaching, not through killing.

Moral courage is nurtured by gentle physical movement, which gives you confidence in yourself. The training and preparation to become a teacher of spiritual swordsmanship is the same as that for the martial arts. The only difference is in the way the goal is achieved. There is no doubt that the world needs help from capable people. Those who wish to offer help through spiritual and peaceful means must have the moral courage of knights of old. Those who act in what looks like evil ways simply do not understand the subtle part of life and need to develop themselves more.

Actually, if you were to kill someone whom you think is an evil person, you would kill only the body; the energy cannot be killed. Rather than trying to kill something that can't be killed, we need to improve and change any environment that fosters the growth of evil. Thus, it is better to leave the body of a so-called evil doer alive, and work in positive ways toward transforming the sociocultural environment. This is the new direction of the school of the spiritual swordsman. For this purpose, a new type of martial art and weapon exercises were developed.

The Power of the Invisible Sword
Is the Power of Your Own Spirit
(I)

Certain physical practices can be used to attain spiritual development, however, if you learn the skills but not the spirit, then you are not yet a student of the School of Spiritual Swordsmanship. This is why I am careful when I teach the skill. At the same time, I need to point out the direction or goal of its origin, which is to help other people develop themselves spiritually.

Thank you for your interest in learning this art. Always remember that it is only for your self-protection. You do not have the right to judge others and use the skill against them.

(II)

When I was practicing Traditional Chinese Medicine in Taiwan, I taught *T'ai Chi* movement. At that time, *T'ai Chi* was taught as a martial art. If you are in the business of teaching martial arts and wish to attract students, you need good achievement or no one will recognize you as a teacher. I was doing quite well in martial arts, but my livelihood came from my medical practice.

One day, an older student who came from northeastern China brought a precious sword from his hometown. It had belonged to someone else, and he had received it as a gift. He was the manager of a big factory who had good business training. I taught him internal *Chi Kung (Chi Gong)* to increase his health, and he gave the sword to me as a gift. I protected it well, but it still needed some special care to prevent it from becoming rusty.

One noon, I wished to clean the sword, so I pulled it from its sheath. I should not have done that at noontime, but I was busy, and that was the only free time I had. The sheath was hard to remove, so I needed to use some force to take the sword out. I used not only force but also the power of my mind. Just as I pulled out the sword, a big rat who was hurt by this somewhat intense energy fell down from the ceiling. It had died on the spot and had no apparent wound in its body. It was hurt by the energy. Friends jokingly described the rat as the evil spirit that happened to hide in my ceiling wishing to steal my energy.

This experience proved to me that the mythology of a good sword's spiritual power is possible. Because I do not have any enemies, my sword has never killed anybody, but that occasion proved that the sword has spiritual power. The sword is power, and the power is a sword.

I gave that sword to a student before I left Taiwan, because such a thing could not be taken out of the country. I hope he is still taking good care of it.

Many stories have been told about precious swords. Some were said to jump down from the wall on which they hung to respond to their master and kill an enemy, or they would make a noise to warn of intruders.

The higher level of spiritual sword was not made of metal, but of personal spiritual energy. Such a sword could kill evil and protect its master's personal spiritual essence.

(III)

Master Lu, Tung Ping of the Tang Dynasty (618-906 C.E.), and Master Tsan, San Fong who came after him, both achieved the art and virtue that belonged to the School of Spiritual Swordsmanship. They also belonged to the School of Golden Immortal Medicine which is the practice of internal and external alchemy.

The School of Spiritual Swordsmanship and the School of

Golden Immortal Medicine are both heritages of the Integral Way. The internal school is an entirely spiritual practice. It is different from the external school, which develops physical energy for fighting. The ancient sages used physical movement to guide students to learn the limitation of physical strength, and thus lead them into spiritual practice.

Physical movement is a tool for spiritual training. Because spirit itself has no form or shape, it cannot be controlled without a certain physical form, shape or movement. For most people, spiritual practice is just the practice of mind through reading, recitation, chanting or prayer. Generally, they do not consider that spiritual practice comes through being. In the Integral Way, spiritual practice is also the practice of being. Whatever you do, you become. Thus, doing any of the gentle movements is more beneficial and direct than praying. Prayer is external, because a person prays to external beings, by chanting or reciting a *sutra* or whatever. The Integral Way goes directly to your life being and is directly involved with your life movement.

(IV)

New generations continue the spirit of the Spiritual Swordsman by accepting the invisible sword as a metaphor for cultivating and refining their spirit. Let me explain further.

In Chinese culture, the materials used to make a sword need to go through a long process. A great quantity of pig iron must be refined to produce the quality of steel fit for a sword. In ancient times, a sword was usually made by using water and fire. Metal was heated in the fire, shaped, and then put into water to be cooled. This process was repeated over and over again. It took many repetitions to make a sword so refined and sharp that it could split a hair, and making a sword turn out well required great spiritual attention. It was not a simple procedure, sometimes it took years. Some swords were so finely made that they were not only very sharp, but were also very flexible. They could be bent back or curved, but when released would return to their original straightness.

This process is similar to the process of spiritual cultivation. The development of human spirits is similar to the process of alternating heat and cold. Through the heat of fire and cold of water, a person's soul becomes firm and right to the point. The water and the fire in a person's life are the troublesome circumstances and experiences through which one learns to improve oneself and develop an indestructible and undefeatable character.

Spiritual swordsmanship is not based on the sharpness of cutting with a physical sword, but upon the greater power of righteousness and harmony. This again describes the difference between the internal and external schools.

(V)

When I was a teenager, most people in China did not like to leave their home town. However, an elder encouraged me to do so. He said, "If you wish to face the entire world, your hometown is not the place to stay. Only by meeting trials and ordeals will you become mature. A person of the Way makes all towns his home, all nations his nation and all people his kin. The way to achieve oneself in the Way is by first learning to give up all easily obtained support from others, then to create your own life by meeting all possible difficulties. The strongest spirit can only be realized by going through the overly heated fire and overly cold ice of life circumstances. If one can rise above them, one has mastered life."

When I was young, I was not smart enough to be a student of spiritual immortality. Instead, I was attracted by physical arts and the great swordsmen in stories. It was not until later that I deeply appreciated the type of spiritual swordsmanship described by Chuang Tzu in his story of the butcher who used his knife for nineteen years without sharpening it. It had no nicks or dents because of the butcher's refinement and skill in the use of the blade. That was a great education.

Refinement is something that we need to learn and use in our daily lives. This is especially true today because of the interdependence of many elements of modern life. People live by supporting one another. A cooperative spirit and a willingness to help are needed.

A refined human soul can do its necessary work in the world and return to its firmness, straightness, earnestness and righteousness. Just as a sword is usually protected by a sheath, the human soul is protected by the physical body.

The reward of teaching is the spiritual development of all people. My spiritual teaching comes from my achievement in swordsmanship, while my teaching of physical arts is from my spiritual learning. My private joy is practicing the arts.

Section 2: Cosmic Tour *Ba Gua Zahn*

Master Ni performed Cosmic Tour *Ba Gua Zahn* at the New Year Celebration and Open House of Yo San University of Traditional Chinese Medicine in Santa Monica, California. Dr. Maoshing Ni read the following description of Cosmic Tour:

The eight natural energies are typically called *Ba Gua* in Chinese, and are represented by the symbols of the sky, lake, fire, thunder, wind, ocean, mountain and earth.

This movement, called Cosmic Tour, is one of the energy conducting exercises for improving health and longevity. It is done in a circular pattern, and all of its movements take place within the circle.

The first section is the movement of sky energy. It symbolizes the continual revolution of the sun, moon and stars, the movements of the clouds, and mimics the activities of our winged friends, the birds.

The second section is the action of lake energy. It symbolizes the gentle, graceful movement of water, such as joyful rain or a beautiful lake, and represents the pure energy of young maidens.

The third section shows the influence of fire energy. This may be symbolized by the transforming activity of a warming fire in a cold house or the brightness of an autumn bonfire in the darkness.

The fourth section demonstrates the animation of thunder energy. It symbolizes the freedom of thunder to reach out in all directions and give a glimpse of illumination to all people.

The fifth section is related to the energy of the wind. It depicts the varied expressions of the air and the changes in the wind's power from a soft, gentle blowing to the rapid rush and powerful force of a tornado.

The sixth section represents the energy of the ocean, which stirs the vitality of all lives. It symbolizes the great water from which all lives obtain their source. This movement offers an experience of the waves of the ocean and its great power, the vastness of the tides, and the joy of the multitude of water lives such as fish and aquatic plants.

The seventh section is the movement of mountain energy. The mountain holds abundant life energy which manifests through gentle stability and steadfastness. It also represents a young gentleman, full of life, who has these same qualities.

The eighth section symbolizes earth energy. Mother earth is receptive to the influence of heavenly energies, and in turn offers her constant support and nurturance to all earthly lives.

Thus, Cosmic Tour Movement begins with the division of eight trigrams, as symbolized by the *ba gua* octahedron (see diagram in Chapter 13), and contains the sixty-four hexagrams of the *I Ching*. The order of the eight main sections follows the mystical Nine-House System that was used in ancient spiritual practices and was developed into the movement of Cosmic Tour much later.

The *Ba Gua* octahedron can be arranged in two ways: pre-Heaven and post-Heaven. The octahedron of pre-Heaven represents the spiritual order of nature, while the octahedron of post-Heaven presents natural functions of manifest nature. The *Ba Gua* itself originated from the ancient spiritual practice called "Walking on the Seven Stars" which is like the crown of the whole set of Cosmic Tour movements, but which is an entirely different level of exercise.

The deeper spiritual practices were mostly inherited from the Great Yu who developed or rather discovered the post-Heaven arrangement of natural energies. The legend says that the arrangement was seen in the whorls on the back of a horse that emerged from the Lu River.

Pre-Heaven refers to the stage of pre-existence, while post-Heaven refers to the stage in which there are people and in which human consciousness attributes particular meaning to things. Thus, my personal understanding is that the pre-Heaven arrangement is more related to the natural environment, whereas the post-Heaven arrangement focuses on the interplay of opposites. Together, they comprise a sense of natural completeness.

My book, *The Natural Paradigm of the Universe*, contains more information about these two ancient diagrams, the post-Heaven being based on *Lu Su* and pre-Heaven on *Hu Tu*.

Chapter 15

Begin to Practice

Instructions for the Simplified Forms of Physical Arts

There are different ways to maintain the form of life.
Students of life know to nurture the subtle essence.
Students of death only know how to excite the body.
Balance comes from caring for both the body and the essence.
- Lao Tzu

Simplified Cosmic Tour *Ba Gua Zahn*:
Merry-Go-Round
Adapted from *Power of Natural Healing* by Hua-Ching Ni

I will begin with a basic description of the movement. To do Merry-Go-Round, you need an open piece of ground. It is a circular movement that can be done in either a clockwise or counterclockwise direction. The circle is usually 28 steps, which symbolize the twenty-eight constellations. You do not need to draw the circle on the ground, just approximate it. The circle can be big or small, but if it is too big, your energy will be too scattered, and if it is too small, your energy will be too tight. Once you start to do it, you do not need to measure it step by step. If you measure it, your relaxation and flexibility will decrease and you will not benefit.

Start by visualizing the image of a flying bird or a swimming fish. Imagine the vast sky and ocean providing you with total freedom. That feeling of freedom makes you know that you are a life being that can extend its energy to unite with that freedom. Never be hurried, but do it at a speed at which you feel comfortable. Do it anytime. When you do it, feel like you are in a deep, grassy meadow, so your walking has a little obstruction or energy field. You could also feel like you are wading in a stream or walking in deep snow. Your main soul is in your head, but because there are channels that connect the top of the body to the feet, the soul is connected to the earth by walking.

As when doing any *T'ai Chi* movement, be well-rooted as you walk. That is, transfer your weight totally with each step and feel your connection with the earth. Be sure to breathe through the nose and bring the breath low into the abdomen. Keep the spine erect or slightly bowed as previously discussed. The arms can be spread open like a bird's wings. You can have one hand in front and one in back, or both hands in back. There are many postures.

Go in one direction, and when you feel you have had enough, turn around and go in the other direction. Relax and enjoy yourself; be creative. Create the wonderful feeling of a free flying bird, or the wonderful feeling of a small child pretending that it is a bird. When you are doing the Merry-Go-Round, always keep moving around the circle.

There are three possible ways to position your legs as you walk: legs not overly bent, like ordinary walking, which will keep you higher; legs bent slightly, which will put you in a middle position; and legs quite bent, which will make you lower. I believe it is preferable to be in a natural position. The lower position is for people with a martial arts purpose. If you are too high, the energy will not center as well as if you are a little seated. Centering well means to be centered in the lower abdomen, the Lower *Tan Tien*.

In the circle movement, there are only two possibilities: one way is with the left hand inside the circle, and the other way is with the right hand inside the circle.

There is also the variable of where to position your hands and arms. I will give the postures one by one.

Continue to do each movement until you feel it is enough or

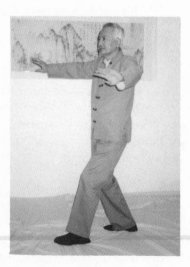

are tired of one hand position, then change to another. Do not change too often. Each hand position stimulates the brain differently, providing a healthy stimulation to the body systems, the internal organs and the brain. This has a good effect on your general health and longevity.

First position: stretch both hands out to the sides at shoulder level, palms down, and keep them open like the wings of a flying bird (Figure 1).

Figure 1

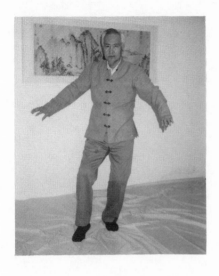

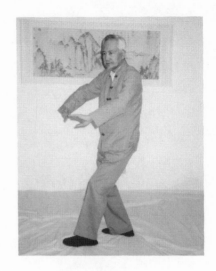

Figure 2   Figure 3

Second position: put your hands some distance from the body, outstretched at the sides around 30 degrees below the horizontal. The arms should not be totally straight; the hands are bent at the wrists with the palms facing and parallel to the ground (Figure 2).

Third position: move both arms in front of the body, about 45 degrees below the horizontal. The fingers of each hand are pointing at each other, with the palms facing downward toward the ground (Figure 3).

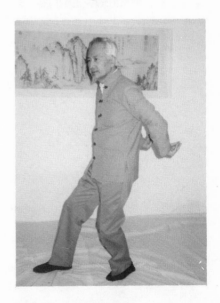

Figure 4

Fourth position: form each hand like a beak by putting the fingertips and the thumb together in a point and then bending the wrist forward so that the "beak" is

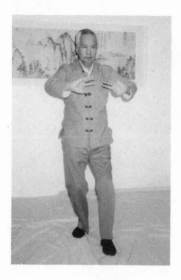

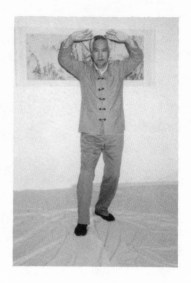

Figure 5	Figure 6

aiming at the elbow and the hands are down. Then swing both of your straight arms behind your back, so that you are like a bird flying (Figure 4).

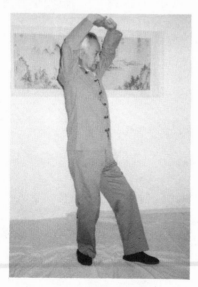

Figure 7

Fifth position: hold your hands up with the fingers pointing to one another. The palms face forward. The arms are not quite fully outstretched horizontally in front of the body at chest height, with the elbows pointing out (Figure 5).

Sixth position: raise your hands from chest level in the fifth position to around 45 to 60 degrees above the horizontal. This places the hands almost over your head, with the fingers pointing toward one another, palms facing down. (Figure 6).

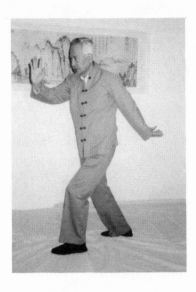 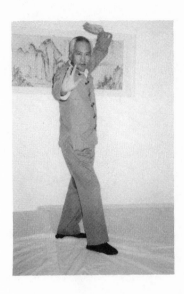

Figure 8   Figure 9

Seventh position: raise the hands, with the palms facing the sky, the same as the sixth position, but straighten your arms upward (Figure 7).

Eighth position: with the chest facing forward, hold the arm inside the circle in front of the center of the chest, with the hand bent upward at the wrist so that the thumb is toward you, and the fingers are pointing to the sky. The arm outside the circle is behind you with its hand bent forward, thumb toward you and fingers pointing toward the sky like a willow palm. The arm should be straight, but not stiff (Figure 8).

Ninth position: point the palm of the hand inside the circle toward the center, and raise the hand on the outside of the circle over the head, with its palm facing the sky. The arm inside the circle is slightly bent and extended toward the center of the circle, while the arm outside the circle is directly over the top of the head with the palm facing the sky (Figure 9).

Tenth position: hold both hands in front of the body with elbows bent at shoulder level. Palms are facing one another about four

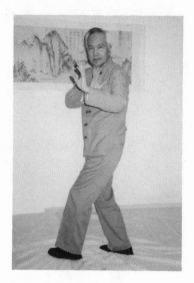

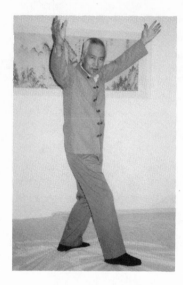

Figure 10   Figure 11

inches apart, but one hand is slightly farther in front than the other (Figure 10). The fingertips of both hands face the sky. You can switch back and forth which hand is in front of the other every few steps, but not too quickly.

Eleventh position: raise the arms up in front of you with palms open, as if you were going to receive some energy from Heaven. The palms somewhat face each other, with the arms slanted away from the body, about 30 degrees above the horizontal (Figure 11).

These are the basic eleven hand and arm positions. You can also change direction from clockwise to counterclockwise around the circumference of the circle. You can move clockwise in one posture, then move counter-clockwise in the same posture. I think whatever graceful, natural way you find to change directions is the best. In ancient times, these turns were programmed to be either simple or complicated, but the point is to make a turn, so use your creativity and see what graceful ways you can come up with.[11]

---

[11]*For a further description of Merry-Go-Round, please see Hua-Ching Ni's book* Power of Natural Healing. *For more detailed practice, please see his book* Cosmic Tour Ba Gua Zahn *and its companion videotape.*

First Movement of Crane Style *Chi Gong*
Adapted from *Crane Style Chi Gong and Its Therapeutic Effects*
by Dr. Daoshing Ni

1. Uniting with the Six Directions and the Return of *Chi*

Generally speaking, Uniting with the Six Directions indicates the communication of man with the energies of the six directions. Man is in the center communicating with East, West, North, South, Heaven and Earth. The purpose of this group of movements is to let our internal energy communicate with the environment, take in the good energy of the universe, and expel our bad energy, or bad *chi*. The flow of *chi* in the channels of our body is harmonized with the directional energy channels of the environment. The external energy of the six directions is then harmonized with the six *Zhang* organs and six *Fu* organs in your body. In Chinese medicine, the six *Zhang* organs are heart, spleen, liver, lung, kidney and pericardium; the six *Fu* organs are small intestine, large intestine, stomach, gall bladder, urinary bladder and *Sanjiao*. *Sanjiao* consists of the three body cavities: the chest cavity, the gastric cavity and the abdominal cavity. These organs have different functions in Chinese medicine than in Western medicine. Harmony and balance between the energy of the six directions and the *Zhang-Fu* organs assures proper functioning of these organs. After Uniting with the Six Directions, we need to return our external *chi* back to the lower abdomen through the point *Du* 20 (Hundred Meeting Point or *Baihui*). Storing the external good *chi* in the lower abdomen can increase our energy and enhance balanced metabolism. The movements of the Return of *Chi* therefore increase blood circulation, strengthen metabolic function, and increase vitality.

There are a total of nine crane-like movements in this section. They are as follows:

1. Preparation: Stand naturally and face South, with toes pointing forward. Feet are shoulder-width apart. The arms rest naturally at the sides. Stand quietly. The tip of the tongue touches the upper palate inside the mouth just behind the teeth. The facial muscles are relaxed. Eyes look straight ahead. The mind is clear as the blue sky without worries. Relax the body from head to toe. Let the *chi* sink down to the Lower *Tan Tien* in the lower abdomen.

Imagining yourself as a crane is the key to all movements. (Fig. 1.)

2. Raising the Wings: Guide the *chi* in the Lower *Tan Tien* to the perineum; raise it up the spine to the point *Du* 14 (Large Vertebra or *Daizhui*) between the shoulders; then direct it through the arms to the point *P* 8 (Labor House or *Laogong*) in the palms. With palms facing downward, slowly raise the arms straight forward to shoulder level. Turn the hands upward at a 90-degree angle to the forearms so the fingers point up and palms face forward. Push out and then retract softly. Inhale when retracting, exhale when pushing out. Push and retract three times. (Figs. 2-5.)

3. Opening the Wings: Loosen up the wrists and, inhaling, open the arms out to the sides at shoulder level. Then turn the hands upward at a 90-degree angle to the forearms so that fingers point up, palms facing East and West. Exhale. Push out and then retract softly three times. Inhale when retracting, exhale when pushing out. (Figs. 6-8.)

4. Closing the Wings: Arms sink down to about 20 degrees from the sides; then push arms back 45 degrees from the sides and raise the heels. Inhale when doing this movement. (Figs. 9-11).

5. Contorting the Wings: With the arms as in Position 4, bend the wrists backward with fingers and thumbs together like claws, then throw the arms forward under the armpits to the front with fingers open, palms facing the sky. While doing this movement, the raised heel hits the ground forcefully with the knees bent. Exhale as the arms are thrown forward. (Figs. 12-13.)

The purpose is to expel stale, pathological, waste *chi* out of the body through the fingers, and retain the clean *chi*. The heel hitting the ground forcefully causes the rise of internal *chi* to promote smooth circulation of *chi* in the body. This movement unites with North.

6. Holding the *Chi* into the Vertex of the Head: Inhale and slowly raise the arms, palms facing upward as if holding a big balloon. Raise arms above the head with the point *P* 8 (Labor House or *Laogong*) of the palms facing the point *Du* 20 (Hundred Meeting or *Baihui*) at the vertex of the head. Transfer the *chi* from *P* 8 to *Du* 20 by exhaling. (Figs. 14-16.)

This movement is to transfer the *chi* to the point *Du* 20 where the *chi* will communicate with Heaven in the next movement.

7. <u>Uniting with Heaven</u>: Inhaling, cross the fingers just above the top of the head with the palms facing the vertex. Then, exhaling, with the legs straight, turn the hands with palms facing the sky and push upward. Bend the knees and return the hands to just above the head, turning the palms downward. With the legs bent, use the vertebras of the neck as an axle and move the head in a circular motion from left to right. Then push upward with the legs straight and palms facing the sky. Bend the knees again and do the same motion on the vertebras of the upper back, and then the lower back. When doing this on the vertebras of the lower back, with hands pushing upward, the back also stretches downward. (Fig. 17)

The purpose of this movement is to loosen the vertebras and open up the channel of the spine which in Chinese Medicine is the *yang* Governing Channel. In the universe, Heaven is *yang* and Earth is *yin*; above our body is *yang* and below is *yin*. Transfer the *chi* from *P* 8 (Labor House or *Laogong*) to *Du* 20 (Hundred Meeting or *Baihui*) and then bring it down to harmonize with both the *yin* and *yang* energy of the body. The palms are turned upward to receive the *yang chi* from Heaven and integrate our body's *yang chi* with the *yang chi* of the universe. The purpose is to use the external *yang chi* to tonify our *yang chi*. When the vertebras are moved, the Governing Channel is activated with *yang chi* which ascends to *Du* 20 and meets with the *yang chi* of the universe. When the vertebras are relaxed, the *yin chi* descends and there is a *yin-yang* balance in the body.

8. <u>Uniting with Earth</u>: The legs are straight and the hands are still together, fingers interlaced. Exhaling, bend forward with the hands pushing straight downward in the center. Raise the hands up to the level of the knees and then push down to the left. Raise up again and push down the right. Push down with exhalation and raise with inhalation. (Fig. 18.)

The Earth is abundant in *yin chi*. This movement integrates internal and external *yin chi* through the point *K* 1 (Bubbling Spring or *Yongchuan*) in the middle of the soles. Its purpose is to use the external *yin chi* to tonify the internal *yin chi*.

9. <u>Return of *Chi*</u>: Transfer the center of gravity to the right leg and lift up the arms. Place the left foot forward, and at the same time raise the left hand to eye level in front of the body with the left palm facing diagonally upward while bringing the right hand down to the side of the right lower abdomen with the right palm facing upward. Inhale when doing the above motion. While exhaling, the head turns slightly to the left side; the eyes look at the point *P* 8 (Labor House or *Laogong*) on the left palm. (Figs. 19-21.)

Turn the head back upright and raise the left arm up higher with the point *P* 8 (Labor House or *Laogong*) facing *Du* 20 (Hundred Meeting or *Baihui*). Exhale the *chi* out *P 8* and inhale into *Du* 20. Do this three times.

Exhaling, bring left hand with the palm facing downward passing beside the left ear to the level of the lower *tan tien*. (Fig. 22.)

Move the center of gravity to the left leg and perform the same motion as above for the right side. (Fig. 23-25)

Shift the body weight to the right leg and bring the left leg forward so that the feet are shoulder-width apart and knees bent. With palms down, bring the arms back slightly behind the body. Then moving them out from the sides, describe a forward arc, bringing the hands forward with the arms extended. Then bring the arms slightly back toward the body with the palms facing the lower *tan tien* and finger tips facing each other. (Fig. 26-27)

As mentioned in the beginning, Return of *Chi* is a process of returning the external *chi* back to the Lower *Tan Tien*.

In summary, this section of movements emphasizes Uniting with the Six Directions through the points *P* 8, *Du* 20 and K 1 (Rushing Spring or *Yongchuan*). After a period of practice, the *chi* in every part of the body will intermingle and harmonize, promoting a more balanced energy state which promotes a healthier body.

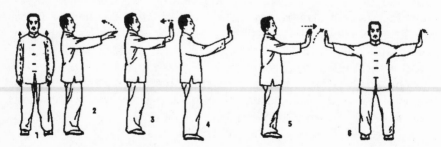

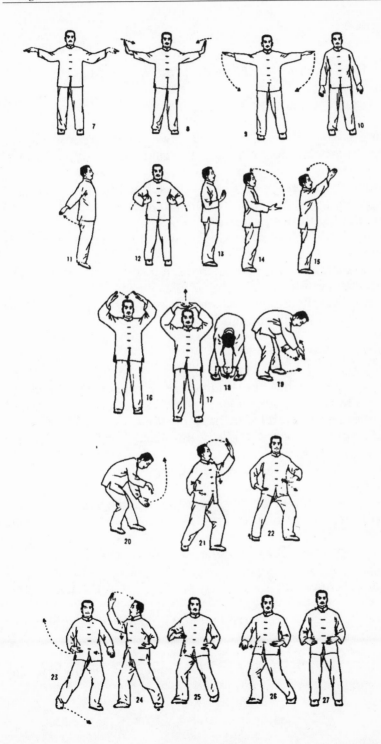

A Selection of *Dao-In* Exercises
Adapted from *Attune Your Body with Dao-In* by Hua-Ching Ni

#2 Immortal Straightening the Leg

Beginning Posture: Lie on back with legs straight. Feet are apart; arms are straight and rest naturally alongside the body, palms up.

1. Inhaling, bend left knee, folding the left leg up to the chest.
2. Clasp bent leg with hands; fingers are interlaced. Body should be relaxed with head on floor.
3. Exhaling, circle foot at ankle 5 times clockwise and 5 times counter-clockwise.
4. Inhaling, straighten the knee so the leg is straight up, perpendicular to the floor.
5. Exhaling, gently and slowly lower the straight leg to the floor and return to the beginning posture.

Instructions for Opposite Side

6. Inhaling, bend right knee, folding the right leg up to the chest.
7. Clasp bent leg with hands; fingers are interlaced. Body should be relaxed and natural with head on floor.
8. Exhaling, circle foot at ankle 5 times clockwise and 5 times counter-clockwise.
9. Inhaling, straighten the knee so the leg is straight up, perpendicular to the floor.
10. Exhaling, gently and slowly lower the straight leg to the floor and return to beginning posture.

Note: This movement may be done once or repeated 3 times.

#17 Immortal Imitating a Lizard Turning to Watch the Dragonfly

Beginning Posture: Sitting crosslegged with hands clasped behind head. Elbows out to side.

1. Exhaling, bend forward at the waist and twist the body to the left, bringing the right elbow down to the center line of the

body, slightly lower than the knees.

2. Inhaling, return to the beginning posture.
3. Exhaling, bend forward at the waist twisting the body to the right, bringing the left elbow to the center line of the body and slightly lower than the knees.
4. Inhaling, return to beginning posture.
5. Exhaling, bend forward at the waist (slightly lower than before) twisting the body to the left, bringing the right elbow to the center line of the body and 3 - 5 inches from the floor.
6. Inhaling, return to beginning posture.
7. Exhaling, bend forward at the waist, twisting the body to the right, bringing the left elbow to the center line of the body 3 - 5 inches from the floor.
8. Inhaling, return to beginning posture.

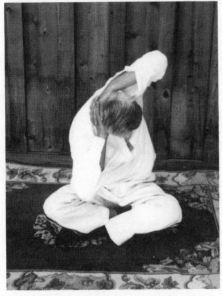

(Dao-In Exercise #17)

9. Exhaling, bend forward at the waist, twisting the body left, bringing the right elbow to the center line of the body and to the floor.
10. Inhaling, return to beginning posture.
11. Exhaling, bend forward at the waist, twisting the body to the right, bringing the left elbow to the center line of the body and to the floor.
12. Inhaling, return to beginning posture.

Note: This movement can only be done in daytime on an empty stomach.

#32 Earth Turning Slowly

Beginning Posture: Sitting crosslegged

1. Place the palms over the kidneys.
2. Massage the area over the kidneys with both palms. Start with the palms on both sides of the spine, circle up, then to the outside, circle down, then return to both sides of spine. Circle 36 times.

Note: This can be done by itself or with the entire set. Persons with kidney weakness should increase the number. It can be done day or night.

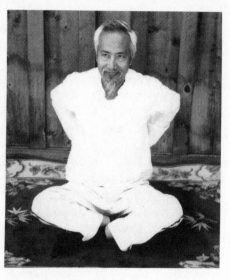

(Dao-In Exercise #32)

#42 Immortal Imitating the Wriggle of the Young Dragon

Beginning Posture: Sitting with left leg straight in front. Right leg bent at the knee with the right foot on floor alongside the left knee, and the right knee pointing up. Arms straight and placed behind the body, palms on the floor, upper body leaning back at a 45-degree angle supported by the arms.

1. Inhaling, lift the body, raising the buttocks as high as possible. Tilt the head back.
2. Exhaling, return to beginning posture.
3. Repeat steps 1 and 2 for a total of 7 times.

Instructions for Opposite Side

Beginning Posture: Sitting with right leg straight in front. Left leg bent at the knee with left foot on floor alongside. Arms straight and placed behind body, palms on floor.

4. Inhaling, lift body, raising buttocks as high as possible. Tilt head back.
5. Exhaling, return to beginning posture.

6. Repeat steps 1 and 2 for a total of 7 times.
7. Still leaning back on arms, place both legs straight in front.
8. Inhaling, lift body, raising buttocks as high as possible. Tilt head back.
9. Exhaling, lower body.
10. Repeat steps 5 and 6 to make a total of 7 times.

Note: This movement should be done with other movements in the daytime.

#33 Immortal Turning the Pulley to Raise the Energy

Beginning Posture: Sitting crosslegged, arms relaxed with hands alongside hips.

1. Circle the right shoulder, from front to back, 36 times.
2. Circle the left shoulder, from front to back, 36 times.

#44 Immortal Holding the Foot to Strengthen the Knee

Beginning Posture: Sitting with left leg straight in front and right leg bent, knee up, right foot close to right buttock. Hands are under right foot, fingers interlocked.

1. Exhaling, straighten the right leg with hands still clasped under foot.
2. Inhaling, return to beginning posture.
3. Repeat steps 1 and 2 for a total of 5 times.

Instructions for Opposite Side

Beginning Posture: sitting with right leg straight in front and left leg bent, knee up, left foot close to left buttock. Hands are under left foot, fingers interlaced.

4. Exhaling, straighten left leg with hands still clasped under foot.
5. Inhaling, return to beginning posture.
6. Repeat steps 4 and 5 for a total of 5 times.

Note: This may be done with the whole set or by itself. Avoid doing this movement at night because it stimulates circulation to the head.

#45 Immortal Bowing to the Rising Sun

Beginning Posture: sitting with both legs straight in front.

1. Exhaling, bend forward at the waist and grasp the top of both feet with the hands.

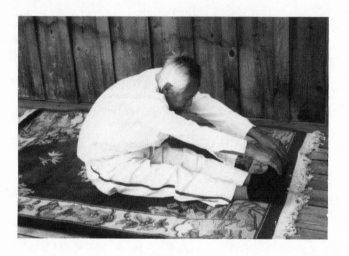

(Dao-In Exercise #46)

2. Inhaling, still holding the feet, raise body up by straightening back slightly and tilt chin up.
3. Exhaling, still holding the feet, bend forward and begin making large circles with the feet; right counter-clockwise and left foot clockwise.
4. Inhaling and exhaling naturally, continue circling the feet 21 times. Then reverse the direction of the circles, right clockwise and left counter-clockwise and circle 21 times.

Note: This should be done along with other movements and can be done at night.

#53 Immortal Doing Eye Acupressure

Beginning Posture: Sitting crosslegged

1. Place the tip of the middle fingers on top of the index fingernails.

2. Press the 3 points on the eyebrows and hold five second each
    a. Inside edge of eyebrow
    b. Middle of eyebrow
    c. Outer corner of eyebrow

3. Repeat step 2 for a total of 3 times.

Note: Press each day to relieve tension.

Simplified Eight Treasures
Adapted from *The Eight Treasures: Energy Enhancement Exercise*
by Dr. Maoshing Ni

Eight Treasures WARM-UP

HOW TO PRACTICE:
Always warm-up before practicing the Eight Treasures. The warm-up may also be done by itself to promote energy circulation at any time during the day. Doing the warm-up may help relieve stress, such as before or after work.

Swinging the Arms - Warming Up the Trunk Area
Let your arms hang down the sides of the body. Relax the neck and shoulder muscles. Initiate a turning movement from the waist and pelvic area to cause your arms to swing. At the end point of each turn, bend the elbows slightly and then relax the arms again through the next turn. Let your loose fists gently pound the area below your waist in front and back, which is called the Lower *Tan Tien*. Continue pounding, gradually moving fists upward toward the navel and then out toward the sides. Continue pounding, gradually moving up the chest and to the shoulders. Gradually backtrack down the same path. Finish at the Lower *Tan Tien*. This movement may be done for two to three minutes.

Raise One Arm While The Other Gently Pounds
Raise one arm out to the front, palm facing down, and close that hand in a loose fist. Use the other loose fist to gently pound, starting at the same side of the lower abdomen as your raised arm. Pound toward the navel, up the center of the chest and then up and out to the shoulder. Turn the raised arm so that the palm is facing the sky, and pound along the inside of the arm to the wrist. Turn the arm over and pound on the outside of the arm from the wrist to the shoulders. Shake both arms down.
  Repeat for other arm.

Lower Back, Thighs and Legs
Pound gently with both hands on the lower back (kidney area). Bending forward at the waist, gradually pound down the outside of the buttocks, thighs, legs and ankles. Then pound up on the

inside of the ankles, legs, thighs and by the crotch area. Alternately bend and then straighten the knees while pounding the top of the legs by the crotch area for a while.

Arms Swing Toward The Back and Jump Up

Swing arms straight behind you several times, allowing the arms to also swing in front of you. Bend your knees when your arms swing forward and straighten them when your arms swing back for several times. Begin to jump up as the arms swing toward the back. Do this several times. Gradually stop the jumping, then the knee bending, and return to a standing position.

Major Joints Rotation

This is a series for rotating the major joints of the body. It is also basically the same as the Eight Treasures movement called "Weeping Willow Shivers In the Early Morning Breeze." The first part is the neck stretch:

Feet shoulder-width apart, gently rotate the head in one direction. Repeat for the other direction. Keep neck muscles relaxed and your eyes closed.

The next part is the pelvic stretch: With your hands over your lower back (kidney area), gently rotate hips in a circular direction. Repeat in the other direction.

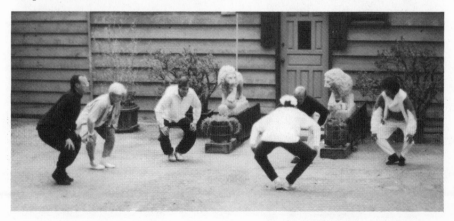

Next are the knee circles: Bend at the waist and rest the hands on the knees. Bend the knees to one side. Move them around to the front, the other side, and behind, making a circle around the feet. For the knees to go in the behind part of each circle, the legs will temporarily straighten. Repeat in the other direction. Return knees to the center.

Move both knees forward and then out to each side, backward and to center, making two small circles. Again, for the backward movement of each circle, the legs will temporarily straighten. Reverse the direction and repeat.

Now you finish with ankle rotation: Lift one foot. Rotate the foot in one direction, then in the other direction. Point your foot; flex your foot. Shake the foot with loose ankle joint. Repeat with the other foot.

Several Simple Movements of the Eight Treasures

Here are several of the more simple movements of the Eight Treasures. The full Eight Treasures works with the entire body, benefiting all the organs, joints, muscles and nervous system. As with the other *chi* exercises we discussed, breathe through the nose from the lower abdomen and keep the tongue curled up against the roof of the mouth. Practice the movements slowly, especially at first, and stay relaxed throughout.

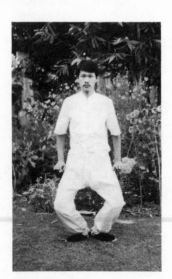

The Dolphin's Fins Pat the Water

This movement is in the first Treasure, which focuses on the organs in the trunk of the body.

Place heels together and toes together. Place your palms on your hips. Rub down the outside of the thighs to the knees and then rub up the inside of the thighs to the waist and circle back to the hips. Repeat several times.

*When the hands are at your waist, turn out the toes as you bring your hands at waist-level to your sides. Then, exhaling, bend the legs (as though sitting with the knees angled to the sides) and lower the hands with palms facing down. Straightening the legs, place the palms on your lower back and rub the thighs once more. Repeat from * several times.

The Great Bird Spreads Its Wings
This movement is in the second treasure; among its purposes are to benefit the lungs.

Place feet more than shoulder-width apart. Bend over at the waist, knees bent slightly, head down and arms hanging down almost touching the ground. Start a gentle rocking motion with your upper body and arms moving front to back, letting your arms swing freely. Straighten up slowly, inhaling, keeping knees bent. Then exhaling, slowly extend arms straight out to the sides, palms facing out and fingers pointing up. Repeat.

Bringing the Stream Back to the Sea
This movement is in the sixth Treasure, and benefits the spine and nervous system.

Bring heels together and hands together. Men place right hand underneath left hand, women place left hand underneath right. Palms face down, thumb of upper hand inside thumb of lower hand and index finger of upper hand covers the lower hand's pinkie joint. Now place hands with palms covering the Lower *Tan Tien*.

Raise the heels and inhale. Keep the spine straight with your chin slightly tucked in. Gently drop the heels and exhale. Repeat several times, no more than 7.

The White Crane Washes Its Wing Feathers
The following movements are in the eighth treasure. Among the primary benefits of the eighth treasure is stronger and healthier kidneys, which are important for life energy.

Stand with feet more than shoulder width apart. Clasp hands together behind the head and bend forward. Twist sideways so

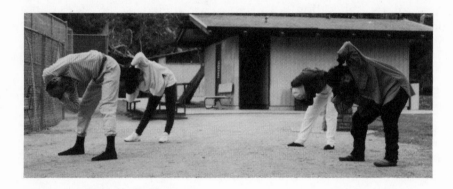

your right elbow is outside your right knee. Look up. Return to the center. Repeat the twist on the other side. Do several on each side.

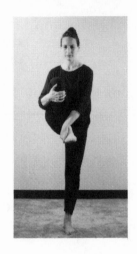

The White Crane Guards the Plum Flower Proudly Standing Alone on the Cold Mountain

Raise your right knee and grasp it with both hands. Gently pull the leg higher and close to the chest several times. Inhale when you pull the leg upward. Slowly release and lower the leg while exhaling. Pull and release a total of three times. Repeat for the other leg.

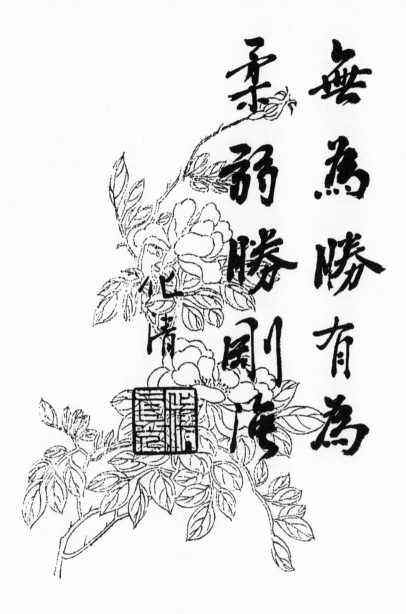

無為勝有為

柔弱勝剛強

The one who does nothing
　　can win over the one who rushes around
　　to do all things.
The one who is gentle
　　can win over the one who is strong.

Chapter 16

Gentle Movement and Quiet Sitting
Are Spiritual Cultivation

1

Treat stillness as movement
and movement as stillness.
Then you can maintain oneness
during either movement or stillness.

2

Find movement in stillness,
and stillness in movement.
You can find self-dissolution in stillness.
You can find self-dissolution in movement.
One who achieves self-dissolution
in movement and in stillness
unites with the Integral Way.

3

By keeping your spirit pure,
you unite with the deep, unchanging truth
and the vast and profound energy ocean.
By not developing partiality toward anyone or anything,
one's life is nurtured along with the Great Nature.

4

Look at things as if they were nothing
and at nothing as if it were something.
By so doing, the mind stays
above beingness and non-beingness,
above things and nothingness.
This is how one unites with all.

5

By emptying the mind and nurturing the chi *of your body,*
you will unite
with the natural spiritual function.
By doing this,
you will reach the creative source of all.

6

Relax your body,
*   repose your mind.*
Be above your body and mind.
Through relaxation and repose,
*   you reach all*
*   and unite with the infinite.*

Achieve this by quiet sitting
*   and gentle movement.*

7

Those who grow from water
*   are happy with water.*
Those who live in water
*   do not know that water exists.*
Fish and the bodies of water
*   - rivers or oceans -*
*   do not know the existence of each other.*

One who realizes the Integral Way
*   travels on turbulent water*
*   as safely as on land,*
*   with no trouble at all.*
This person does not know fear.
This is how to remain untroubled by life.

8

By maintaining empty mindedness and sincerity
*   one can forget the weight of life.*
Follow the middle, balanced way
*   as your sole guidepost to eternal life.*

9

Keep your mind free from fear.
Eliminate all mixed desires and interests.
Protect the serenity of the mind
*   from all intrusion and disturbance.*
Follow the natural rhythm of life.
Carry no worldly worry.
Stop the searching and multiple applications of the mind.
One achieves a good life by self-forgetfulness.

10

A good archer is not nervous while shooting.
In this way, he achieves excellence.
The best swordsman remains calm
*   in a sword fight or fencing match.*
His sword is raised at a slower speed,
*   yet it is first to stop an*
*   impulsive attack from an opponent.*

11

One who faces danger as if there were no danger,
*   and one who faces turbulent water*
*   as if there were no turbulence*
*   has a better chance of overcoming the difficulty.*
One who shoots at a fierce beast
*   as if it were a piece of stone*
*   easily reaches his goal.*

12

Living should be done with the same calmness
*   as practicing archery.*
The secret to enjoying life
*   is first to get rid of fear.*
This can be attained
*   by practicing spiritual cultivation*
*   through gentle movement and meditation.*

For Further Information

It is said that the highest essence of truth is used for examining one's own mind and body.

- Chuang Tzu

The following is a reading list of related materials of interest to practitioners of physical arts, listed by topic. These materials are available through SevenStar Communications.

Breathing

Crane Style Chi Gong, Chapter III, Part 3: "Breathing Regulation."

Power of Natural Healing, Chapter 10: "Breathing Reaches Soul."

Chi

Book of Changes and the Unchanging Truth, Chapter 8: "Natural Energy in Human Life."

Guide to Inner Light, Chapter 2, pages 36-50 and 98-102 for discussion on cultivating *chi.*

Internal Alchemy: The Natural Way to Immortality, "Concluding Instruction," for description of the movement of *chi.*

Life and Teachings of Two Immortals, Volume II: Chen Tuan, Chapter 4: "Internal Energy Conducting and Orbit Circulation."

8,000 Years of Wisdom, Book II, Chapter 60: "The Main Principles of Cultivating *Chi.*"

Chi Kung (Chi Gong)

Crane Style Chi Gong by Dr. Daoshing Ni.

Life and Teachings of Two Immortals, Volume I: Kou Hong, Chapter 4, p. 69-74 for discussion of *chi kung* and *t'ai chi.*

Diet

8,000 Years of Wisdom, Book I, Chapter 35: "Introduction to Diet," Chapter 36: "Foods in General" and Chapter 37: "The Healing Properties of Food."

Tao of Nutrition by Dr. Maoshing Ni and Cathy McNease.

Chinese Vegetarian Delights by Lily Chuang and Cathy McNease.

101 Vegetarian Delights by Lily Chuang and Cathy McNease.

Exercises:

Attune Your Body with Dao-In by Hua-Ching Ni (book and video-tape available).

Cosmic Tour Ba Gua Zahn videotape with instruction book by Hua-Ching Ni (should be available after Summer of 1997).

Crane Style Chi Gong by Dr. Daoshing Ni (book and videotape available).

Eight Treasures videotape and *Eight Treasures: Energy Enhancement Exercise* book, both by Dr. Maoshing Ni.

Gentle Path T'ai Chi videotape with instruction book by Hua-Ching Ni (should be available after Summer of 1996).

Harmony/Trinity T'ai Chi, two videotapes by Maoshing Ni.

Infinite Expansion T'ai Chi videotape with instruction book by Hua-Ching Ni (should be available after Winter of 1996).

Power of Natural Healing, Chapter 9: "Guard Yourself from the Hidden Negative Elements" for spiritual practices and description of Merry-Go-Round.

Self-Healing Chi Gong videotape by Maoshing Ni.

Sky Journey T'ai Chi videotape with instruction book by Hua-Ching Ni (should be available after Spring of 1997).

Health and Healing:

Chinese Herbology by Dr. Maoshing Ni.

Crane Style Chi Gong, Chapter 1: "Chi Gong as a Medical Therapy."

Tao, the Subtle Universal Law, Chapter 3: "The Human Body and Universal Law" and Chapter 4: "The Art of Preserving Health."

Power of Natural Healing by Hua-Ching Ni.

Martial Arts

8,000 Years of Wisdom, Book II, Chapter 54: "Self-Improvement through Martial Arts."

Meditation

Attune Your Body with Dao-In, Chapter 8, pages. 94-106.

Enlightenment: Mother of Spiritual Independence, Chapter 5: "How to Use Meditation to Attain Your Enlightenment."

Eternal Light, Chapter 10: "Guidance for Deep Meditation."

Life and Teachings of Two Immortals, Volume I: Kou Hong, Chapter 3: "Instruction for Good Meditation."

Life and Teachings of Two Immortals, Volume II: Chen Tuan, Chapter 3: "Essential Guidelines for Meditation and Sleeping Meditation."

Story of Two Kingdoms, "Taoist Indoor Meditation," pages 106 - 111.

Mind

Key to Good Fortune by Hua-Ching Ni.

Mysticism: Empowering the Spirit Within by Hua-Ching Ni.

Workbook for Spiritual Development of All People, Chapter 3: "Work to Improve the Quality of Your Mind."

Practitioners of *T'ai Chi* Movement:

Life and Teachings of Two Immortals: Volume I, Kou Hong by Hua-Ching Ni.

Life and Teachings of Two Immortals: Volume II, Chen Tuan by Hua-Ching Ni.

Esoteric Tao Teh Ching for information on the life of Lao Tzu.

Spiritual Classics:

Attaining Unlimited Life (The Book of Chuang Tzu) by Hua-Ching Ni.

The Book of Changes and the Unchanging Truth by Hua-Ching Ni.

Complete Works of Lao Tzu by Hua-Ching Ni, containing the *Tao Teh Ching* and the *Hua Hu Ching*.

Esoteric Tao Teh Ching by Hua-Ching Ni.

Spiritual Practices:

Awaken Your Life Spirit With Complete Meditation by Hua-Ching Ni.

Eternal Light by Hua-Ching Ni.

Gentle Path of Spiritual Progress by Hua-Ching Ni.

Power of Natural Healing by Hua-Ching Ni.

Story of Two Kingdoms by Hua-Ching Ni.

Taoist View of the Universe and the Immortal Realm by Hua-Ching Ni.

Workbook for Spiritual Development of All People by Hua-Ching Ni.

T'ai Chi Movement

Tao, the Subtle Universal Law, Chapter 5: "*T'ai Chi Chuan*, Universal Law and the Law of Individual Being" and Chapter 6: "The Application and Practice of *T'ai Chi Chuan*."

Power of Natural Healing, Chapter 7: "Discussion about Eight Treasures, *Chi Gong* and *T'ai Chi* Movement" and Chapter 8: "Visual Energy Connects with Internal Movement."

Glossary

Note: In this book, the words "physical arts," "gentle movement," "*Chi Kung (Chi Gong)*" and "*T'ai Chi* movement" are sometimes used interchangeably to describe physical *chi* exercise.

Ba Gua: Eight *gua* or trigrams, or an arrangement of the eight trigrams. Also may refer to Cosmic Tour *Ba Gua Zahn* (also expressed in Chinese as *Pa Kua Chang),* an exercise done in a circular movement.

Book of Changes: See also *I Ching*. The legendary classic *Book of Changes* or the *I Ching* is recognized as the first written book of wisdom. Leaders and sages throughout history have consulted it as a trusted advisor which reveals the appropriate action in any circumstance.

Chen Tuan, Master: The "sleeping sage" who refreshed *T'ai Chi* philosophy, living circa 885-989 C.E. at the beginning of the Sung Dynasty.

Chi (also spelled *Qi* or *Ki*): *Chi* is the vitality or life energy of the universe and resides within each living being. In humans, it provides the power for our movements of body and mind, immune system, and all organ functions.

Chi Kung (also spelled *chi gong* or *qi gong*): Translated literally as energy work, energy exercise, or breathing exercise. A set of breathing, movement and/or visualization exercises for strengthening and balancing the *chi* or vital force, relaxing the mind, maintaining health and curing disease. It can be static (no movement) or dynamic (with movement). It is usually a single exercise or a small group of exercises practiced separately or together.

Chuang Tzu: A Taoist sage who lived around 275 B.C. and wrote an influential book called *Chuang Tzu.*

Conception (*Ren*) channel: Expressed in Chinese as *Ren Mai* or *Jen Mo.* Also translated as Conception Vessel. It is the main *yin* channel and is one of the eight extraordinary channels; occurs as a single channel on the midline of the front of the body.

Dao-In: A series of *chi kung* type movements traditionally used for conducting physical energy. The ancients discovered that *Dao-In* exercise solves problems of stagnant energy, increases health, lengthens one's years, and provides support for cultivation and higher achievements of spiritual immortality.

_Du 20_ (Hundred Meeting) point: Expressed in Chinese as _Bai Hui,_
Bai Hwei or _Pai Hui_. Also called All Meeting, Thousand-Meeting, the
Vertex, or the Crown Point. It is the meeting point of all the _Yang_
channels which traverse the head. It is located on the top midline of
the head, in line with the tops of the ears. _Du_ 20 is very close to the so-
called "soft spot" of an infant. Through _Du_ 20, we make our connection
with Heavenly energy.

Eight Treasures: A form of _Dao-In_, a type of internal exercise or _chi_
kung patterned after natural movements.

External School: A school of physical training which teaches regular
martial arts such as how to use and increase one's fighting skill and
force. Emphasizes muscular development and strength.

Feng Shui: Geomancy, arrangement of the energy relationships of
one's environment which seeks to make their effect more supportive
of life.

_Fu_ Organs: In Traditional Chinese Medicine, the so-called "hollow
organs," consisting of the small intestine, large intestine, stomach, gall
bladder, urinary bladder and triple heater (_San Jiao_). Paired with the
Zhang organs.

Fu Shi: Ancient one who developed a "line system" to express the
principle of appropriateness, which is the basis of the present _I Ching_.

Governing _(Du)_ Channel: Also expressed in Chinese as _Du Mao_ or _Tu_
_Mo_, and in English as Governing Vessel. One of the eight extraordinary channels, occurs as a single channel on the midline of the back of
the body. It "governs" the _yang_ energy of the body.

Harmony/Trinity _T'ai Chi_ Movement: A _t'ai chi_ style comprising movements of three popular styles, Wu, Chen and Yang.

Heavenly Eye Point: Also called the Upper _Tan Tien._ Expressed in
Chinese as _Tien Mu._ Located on the lower forehead one third of the
distance from the point between the eyebrows up to the front hairline.
This is an "extra point," not associated with a channel.

Hui Neng, Master: Sixth patriarch of the Buddhist tradition and father
of Zen Buddhism. An example of a person of ordinary birth who

achieved himself to become a "spiritual diamond."

I Ching: A method of divination which uses the 64 hexagrams originated by Fu Shi. Information about the hexagrams was recorded in a book by the same name which is translated into English as *Book of Changes.*

Integral Way (or the Way, or Tao): The way of knowing, doing and being. The true spiritual achievement of the ancients. Realizing the *t'ai chi* principle of harmony and balance in life.

Internal School: An approach to physical training which teaches physical movement for health and physical education to refine individual energy. Emphasizes internal energy development and refinement.

Jing (Ching or *Tsing):* The gross or "raw" level of energy; can be refined to *chi.*

Jung Yun Yuan Mang: A principle to follow in *t'ai chi* practice which means "full development is attained in movement."

K1 (Rushing Spring) point: Expressed in Chinese as *Yong Chuan, Yong Quan,* or *Yung Chuan.* Also translated in English as Bubbling Spring. Located in the depression which appears in the sole of the foot when the toes are curled, approximately on the midline of the foot at the junction of the anterior and middle thirds of the sole. Through *Yong Chuan,* we make our connection to the energy of the earth.

Kou Hong, Master: Also known in Chinese as Pao Poh Tzu or Bao Boh Tzu. Living 283-262 C.E., during the Jing Dynasty. A balanced personality who provides a model of high spirituality.

Lao Tzu: Also expressed in Chinese as Lao Zi, Lao Tze , or Lao Tse. Achieved master who continued the teaching of natural truth. Author of the *Tao Teh Ching* and *Hua Hu Ching.* (Active around 571 B.C.E.)

Lu, Tung Ping, Master: Promoter of later school of spiritual swordsmanship which followed the moral discipline of Mo Tzu.

Meditation: A form of sitting, standing, or walking *chi kung* which develops centeredness to embrace all. Unites the mind with the body and gathers one's energy.

Nei kung: Internal *chi* exercise.

P 8 (Labor House) point: Expressed in Chinese as *Lao Gong*. Also translated in English as House of Labor or Labor Palace. Located in the palm where the tip of the middle finger touches when making a fist.

Pa Kun Dao-In: Another name for the Eight Treasures.

Push Hands: A form of practice in which two people practice together to apply the skills they learned from the *t'ai chi* forms, especially the skill of the soft conquering the strong.

Ren 1 (Yin Meeting): Also expressed in Chinese as *Hui Yin*. An acupuncture point located at the perineum, the point between the genitals and anus.

San Jiao: Translated as Triple Warmer, Three Warmers, or Triple Heater, which are the three cavities in the chest and abdomen.

Sen (shen): Spirit; also the high or pure level of energy, which can be refined from *chi*.

Shao Lin: A style of martial arts originating from the Shao Lin Temple in Hunan province, China, characterized by its discipline.

Shien: An immortal, a spiritually achieved individual.

Shien Jia Ba Duan Jin: Another name for the Eight Treasures.

Six Healing Sounds: Healing practice used on special occasions. Presented in *Voyage Toward the Subtle Light: The Great Path of Universal Awakening.*

T'ai Chi Movement: Also known in Chinese as *T'ai Chi Chuan* or *Tai Ji Quan*. Ancient Chinese exercise for harmonizing body, mind and spirit, whose connected movements somewhat resemble a graceful dance. Consists of many different *chi kung* movements put together sequentially and arranged with the principles given by the *Tao Teh Ching* and *I Ching*.

T'ai Chi Principle: The principle of alternation of opposites, also called the *Yin/Yang* Principle, the Universal Law, or the Law of *T'ai Chi*.

<u>Tao:</u> The invisible, Integral Way. Profound truth of life.

<u>*Tao Teh Ching:*</u> Also expressed in Chinese as *Dao Deh Jing*. An influ-
ential book written by Lao Tzu as an attempt to elucidate Tao, the
subtle truth of life. Considered a classic, it is among the most widely
translated and distributed books in the world.

<u>*Tan Tien (or Dan Tien):*</u> Translated as "field of elixir," this is more an
area than a specific point on the body. It is generically used to refer to
several energy centers of the body where energy is stored: the Upper
Tan Tien or Heavenly Eye Point, the Middle *Tan Tien* or center of the
chest, and the Lower *Tan Tien* or area around four finger-widths below the navel. *Tan tien* also frequently refers specifically to the Lower
Tan Tien.

<u>*Tien Mu:*</u> See Heavenly Eye Point.

<u>Unity *T'ai Chi* Movement:</u> Another name for Harmony/Trinity *T'ai Chi*
Movement.

<u>*Wu Shu:*</u> All styles of martial arts which originated in China and are
characterized by fighting.

<u>*Wu Wei:*</u> The principle of "doing nothing extra" or "inaction in action,"
"doing just enough," "non-doing," or "harmonious action."

<u>*Yin and Yang:*</u> Terms which describe opposites, the two ends of
either pole, or duality. *Yang* relates to the male, outward, active, positive, fiery, energetic side of life or nature of a person. *Yin* relates to the
female, inward, passive, negative, watery, cool, substantial side of life
or nature of a person.

<u>*Yin Yang Kai Huh:*</u> A special term for the *T'ai Chi* Principle. A prin-
ciple to follow in *t'ai chi* practice which means "the principle of rhythmic
alternation."

<u>*Yuen Chi:*</u> Primal, creative energy or original simplicity.

<u>*Zhang* or *Zang* Organs:</u> In Traditional Chinese Medicine, the so-called
"solid organs," consisting of the heart, spleen, liver, lung, kidney, and
pericardium. Paired with the *Fu* organs.

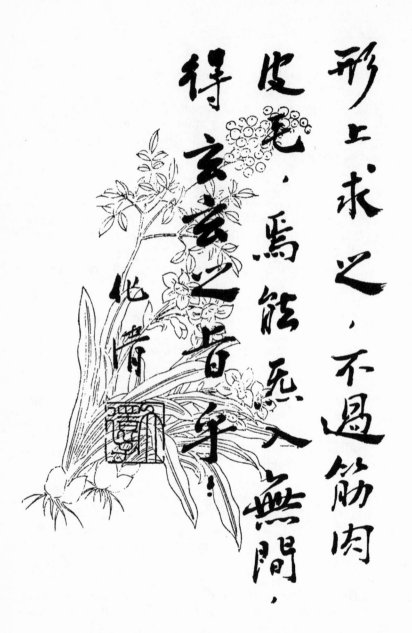

形上求之，不過筋肉
皮毛・焉能无入無間，
得玄玄之旨乎！

化情

If you work on the shallow level,
you only reach the depth of skin and muscles.
You cannot reach the deep subtlety of sen (spirit).

About The Authors

<u>Hua-Ching Ni</u> feels that it is his responsibility to ensure that people receive his message clearly and correctly, thus, he puts his lectures and classes into book form. He does this for the clear purpose of universal spiritual unity.

It will be his great happiness to see the genuine progress of all people, all societies and nations as they become one big harmonious worldly community. This is the goal that inspires him to speak and write as one way of fulfilling his personal duty. The teachings he offers people come from his own growth and attainment.

Hua-Ching Ni began his spiritual pursuit when he was quite young. Although spiritual nature is innate, learning to express it suitably and usefully requires worldly experience and a lot of training. A hard life and hard work have made him deeper and stronger, and perhaps wiser. This is the case with all people who do not yield to the negative influences of life and the world. He does not intend to establish himself as a special individual, as do people in general spiritual society, but wishes to give service. He thinks that he is just one person living on the same plane of life with the rest of humanity.

He likes to be considered a friend rather than have a formal title. In this way he enjoys the natural spiritual response between himself and others who come together in extending the ageless natural spiritual truth to all.

He is a great traveller, and never tires of going to new places. His books have been printed in different languages, having been written at the side of his professional work as a natural healer – a fully trained Traditional Chinese Medical doctor. He understands that his world mission is to awaken people of both east and west, and he supports his friends and helpers as Mentors. All work together to fulfill the world spiritual mission of this time in human history.

<u>Daoshing Ni</u>, C.A., D.O.M., Ph.D. is the author of *Crane Style Chi Gong* and a video of the same name. As a 38th generation medical practitioner in his family, Dr. Ni has received extensive training in Taoist healing arts and medicine from his father, Hua-Ching Ni, and other highly achieved teachers. He has a busy practice of Traditional Chinese Medicine in Santa Monica, California and is the President of Yo San University of Traditional Chinese Medicine where he also teaches Taoist movement classes such as *chi gong* and *t'ai chi* and medical classes.

<u>Maoshing Ni</u>, C.A., D.O.M., Ph.D. is the author of *The Tao of Nutrition, and Chinese Herbology*. He has also authored several audio and video programs on *chi gong, t'ai chi* and Eight Treasures. As a 38th generation medical practitioner in his family, Dr. Ni has received extensive training in Taoist healing arts and medicine from his father, Hua-Ching Ni, and many other achieved teachers. Dr. Ni maintains a busy private practice in Santa Monica, California, where he also instructs at Yo San University of Traditional Chinese Medicine, which he co-founded with his family.

Teachings of the Universal Way by Hua-Ching Ni

NEW RELEASES

Spring Thunder: Awaken the Hibernating Power of Life - Humans need to be periodically awakened from a spiritual hibernation in which the awareness of life's reality is deeply forgotten. To awaken your deep inner life, this book offers the practice of Natural Meditation, the enlightening teachings of Yen Shi, and Master Ni's New Year Message. BSPRI 0-937064-77-7 PAPERBACK, 176 P $12.95

The Eight Treasures: Energy Enhancement Exercise - by Maoshing Ni, Ph. D. The Eight Treasures is an ancient system of energy enhancing movements based on the natural motion of the universe. It can be practiced by anyone at any fitness level, is non-impact, simple to do, and appropriate for all ages. It is recommended that this book be used with its companion videotape. BEIGH 0-937064-55-6 Paperback 208p $17.95

The Universal Path of Natural Life - The way to make your life enduring is to harmonize with the nature of the universe. By doing so, you expand beyond your limits to reach universal life. This book is the third book in the series called *The Course for Total Health*. BUNIV 0-937064-76-9 PAPERBACK, 104P $9.50

Power of Positive Living How do you know if your spirit is healthy? You do not need to be around sickness to learn what health is. When you put aside the cultural and social confusion around you, you can rediscover your true self and restore your natural health. This is the second book of *The Course for Total Health*. BPOWE 0-937064-90-4 PAPERBACK 80P $8.50

The Gate to Infinity - People who have learned spiritually through years without real progress will be thoroughly guided by the important discourse in this book. Master Ni also explains Natural Meditation. Editors recommend that all serious spiritual students who wish to increase their spiritual potency read this one. BGATE 0-937064-68-8 PAPERBACK 208P $13.95

The Yellow Emperor's Classic of Medicine - by Maoshing Ni, Ph.D. The *Neijing* is one of the most important classics of Taoism, as well as the highest authority on traditional Chinese medicine. Written in the form of a discourse between Yellow Emperor and his ministers, this book contains a wealth of knowledge on holistic medicine and how human life can attune itself to receive natural support. BYELLO 1-57062-080-6 PAPERBACK 316P $16.00

Self-Reliance and Constructive Change - Natural spiritual reality is independent of concept. Thus dependency upon religious convention, cultural notions and political ideals must be given up to reach full spiritual potential. The Declaration of Spiritual Independence affirms spiritual self-authority and true wisdom as the highest attainments of life. This is the first book in *The Course for Total Health*. BSELF 0-937064-85-8 PAPERBACK 64P $7.00

Concourse of All Spiritual Paths - All religions, in spite of their surface difference, in their essence return to the great oneness. Hua-Ching Ni looks at what traditional religions offer us today and suggest how to go beyond differences to discover the depth of universal truth. BCONC 0-937064-61-0 PAPERBACK 184P $15.95.

PRACTICAL LIVING

The Key to Good Fortune: Refining Your Spirit - Straighten Your Way *(Tai Shan Kan Yin Pien)* and The Silent Way of Blessing *(Yin Chia Wen)* are the main guidance for a mature, healthy life. Spiritual improvement can be an integral part of realizing a Heavenly life on Earth. BKEYT 0-937064-39-4 PAPERBACK 144P $12.95

Harmony - The Art of Life - The emphasis in this book is on creating harmony within ourselves so that we can find it with other people and with our environment. BHARM 0-937064-37-8 PAPERBACK 208P $14.95

Ageless Counsel for Modern Life - Following the natural organization of the *I Ching*, Hua-Ching Ni has woven inspired commentaries to each of the 64 hexagrams. Taken alone, they display an inherent wisdom which is both personal and profound. BAGEL 0-937064-50-5 PAPERBACK 256P $15.95.

Strength From Movement: Mastering Chi - by Hua-Ching Ni, Daoshing Ni and Maoshing Ni. - *Chi,* the vital power of life, can be developed and cultivated within yourself to help support your healthy, happy life. This book gives the deep reality of different useful forms of *chi* exercise and which types are best for certain types of people. Includes samples of several popular exercises. BSTRE 0-937064-73-4 PAPERBACK WITH 42 PHOTOGRAPHS 256P $16.95.

8,000 Years of Wisdom, Volume I and II - This two-volume set contains a wealth of practical, down-to-earth advice given to students over a five-year period. Volume I includes 3 chapters on dietary guidance. Volume II devotes 7 chapters to sex and pregnancy topics. VOLUME I: BWIS1 0-937064-07-6 PAPERBACK 236P $12.50 • VOLUME II: BWIS2 0-937064-08-4 PAPERBACK 241P $12.50

The Time Is Now for a Better Life and a Better World - What is the purpose of personal spiritual achievement if not to serve humanity by improving the quality of life for everyone? Hua-Ching Ni offers his vision of humanity's dilemma and what can be done about it. BTIME 0-937064-63-7 PAPERBACK 136P $10.95

Spiritual Messages from a Buffalo Rider, A Man of Tao - This book is a collection of talks from Hua-Ching Ni's world tour and offers valuable insights into the interaction between a compassionate spiritual teacher and his students from many countries around the world. BSPIR 0-937064-34-3 PAPERBACK 242P $12.95

Golden Message - by Daoshing and Maoshing Ni - This book is a distillation of the teachings of the Universal Way of Life as taught by the authors' father, Hua-Ching Ni. Included is a complete program of study for students and teachers of the Way. BGOLD 0-937064-36-x PAPERBACK 160P $11.95

Moonlight in the Dark Night - This book contains wisdom on how to control emotions, including how to manage love relationships so that they do not impede one's spiritual achievement. BMOON 0-937064-44-0 PAPERBACK 168P $12.95

SPIRITUAL DEVELOPMENT

Life and Teaching of Two Immortals, Volume 1: Kou Hong - A master who achieved spiritual ascendancy in 363 A.D., Kou Hong was an achieved master in the art of alchemy. His teachings apply the Universal Way to business, politics, emotions, human relationships, health and destiny. BLIF1 0-937064-47-5 PAPERBACK 176P $12.95.

Life and Teaching of Two Immortals, Volume 2: Chen Tuan - Chen Tuan was an achieved master who was famous for the foreknowledge he attained through deep study of the *I Ching* and for his unique method of "sleeping cultivation." This book also includes important details about the microcosmic meditation and mystical instructions from the "Mother of Li Mountain." BLIF2 0-937064-48-3 PAPERBACK 192P $12.95

The Way, the Truth and the Light - *now available in paperback!* - Presented in light, narrative form, this inspiring story unites Eastern and Western beliefs as it chronicles a Western prophet who journeys to the East in pursuit of further spiritual guidance. BLIGH1 0-937064-56-4 PAPERBACK 232P $14.95 • BLIGH2 0-937064-67-X HARDCOVER 232P $22.95

The Mystical Universal Mother - Hua-Ching Ni responds to the questions of his female students through the example of his mother and other historical and mythical women. He focuses on the feminine aspect of both sexes and on the natural relationship between men and women. BMYST 0-937064-45-9 PAPERBACK 240P $14.95

Eternal Light - Dedicated to Yo San Ni, a renowned healer and teacher, and father of Hua-Ching Ni. An intimate look at the lifestyle of a spiritually centered family. BETER 0-937064-38-6 PAPERBACK 208P $14.95

Quest of Soul - How to strengthen your soul, achieve spiritual liberation, and unite with the universal soul. A detailed discussion of the process of death is also included. BQUES 0-937064-26-2 PAPERBACK 152P $11.95

Nurture Your Spirits - Spirits are the foundation of our being. Hua-Ching Ni reveals the truth about "spirits" based on his personal cultivation and experience, so that you can nurture your own spirits. BNURT 0-937064-32-7 PAPERBACK 176P $12.95

Internal Alchemy: The Natural Way to Immortality - Ancient spiritually achieved ones used alchemical terminology metaphorically to disguise personal internal energy transformation. This book offers the prescriptions that help sublimate your energy. BALCH 0-937064-51-3 PAPERBACK 288P $15.95

Mysticism: Empowering the Spirit Within - "Fourteen Details for Immortal Medicine" is a chapter on meditation for women and men. Four other chapters are devoted to the study of 68 mystical diagrams, including the ones on Lao Tzu's tower. BMYST2 0-937064-46-7 PAPERBACK 200P $13.95

Internal Growth through Tao - In this volume, Hua-Ching Ni teaches about the more subtle, much deeper aspects of life. He also points out the confusion caused by some spiritual teachings and encourages students to cultivate internal growth. BINTE 0-937064-27-0 PAPERBACK 208P $13.95

Essence of Universal Spirituality - A review of world religions, revealing the harmony of their essence and helping readers enjoy the achievements of all religions without becoming confused by them. BESSE 0-937064-35-1 PAPERBACK 304P $19.95

Guide to Inner Light - Modern culture diverts our attention from our natural life being. Drawing inspiration from the experience of the ancient achieved ones, Hua-Ching Ni redirects modern people to their true source and to the meaning of life. BGUID 0-937064-30-0 PAPERBACK 192P $12.95

Stepping Stones for Spiritual Success - This volume contains practical and inspiration quotations from the traditional teachings of Tao. The societal values and personal virtues extolled here are relevant to any time or culture. BSTEP 0-937064-25-4 PAPERBACK 160P $12.95.

The Story of Two Kingdoms - The first part of this book is the metaphoric tale of the conflict between the Kingdoms of Light and Darkness. The second part details the steps to self cleansing and self confirmation. BSTOR 0-937064-24-6 HARDCOVER 122P $14.50

The Gentle Path of Spiritual Progress - A companion volume to Messages of a Buffalo Rider. Hua-Ching Ni answers questions on contemporary psychology, sex, how to use the I Ching, and tells some fascinating spiritual legends! BGENT 0-937064-33-5 PAPERBACK 290P $12.95.

Footsteps of the Mystical Child - Profound examination of such issues as wisdom and spiritual evolution open new realms of understanding and personal growth. BFOOT 0-937064-11-4 PAPERBACK 166P $9.50

TIMELESS CLASSICS

The Complete Works of Lao Tzu - The *Tao Teh Ching* is one of the most widely translated and cherished works of literature. Its timeless wisdom provides a bridge to the subtle spiritual truth and aids harmonious and peaceful living. Plus the only authentic written translation of the *Hua Hu Ching*, a later work of Lao Tzu which was lost to the general public for a thousand years. BCOMP 0-937064-00-9 PAPERBACK 212P $13.95

The Book of Changes and the Unchanging Truth - Revised Edition - This version of China's timeless classic *I Ching* is heralded as the standard for modern times. A unique presentation including profound illustrative commentary and details of the book's underlying natural science and philosophy from a world-renowned expert. BBOOK 0-937064-81-5 HARDCOVER 669P $35.00

Workbook for Spiritual Development - This is a practical, hands-on approach for those devoted to spiritual achievement. Diagrams showing sitting postures, standing postures and even a sleeping cultivation. An entire section is devoted to ancient invocations. BWORK 0-937064-06-8 PAPERBACK 240P $14.95

The Esoteric Tao Teh Ching - This totally new edition offers instruction for studying the Tao Teh Ching and reveals the spiritual practices "hidden" in Lao Tzu's classic. These include in-depth techniques for advanced spiritual benefit. BESOT 0-937064-49-1 PAPERBACK 192P $13.95

The Way of Integral Life - The Universal Integral Way leads to a life of balance, health and harmony. This book includes practical suggestions for daily life, philosophical thought, esoteric insight and guidelines for those aspiring to help their lives and the world. BWAYS 0-937064-20-3 PAPERBACK 320P $14.00 • BWAYH 0-937064-21-1 HARDCOVER 320P $20.00.

Enlightenment: Mother of Spiritual Independence - The inspiring story and teachings of Hui Neng, the 6th Patriarch and father of Zen, highlight this volume. Intellectually unsophisticated, Hui Neng achieved himself to become a true spiritual revolutionary. BENLS 0-937064-19-X PAPERBACK 264P $12.50 • BENLH 0-937064-22-X HARDCOVER 264P $22.00.

Attaining Unlimited Life - Most scholars agree that Chuang Tzu produced some of the greatest literature in Chinese history. He also laid the foundation for the Universal Way. In this volume, Hua-Ching Ni draws upon his extensive training to rework the entire book of Chuang Tzu. BATTS 0-937064-18-1 PAPERBACK 467P $18.00; BATTH 0-937064-23-8 HARDCOVER $25.00

The Taoist Inner View of the Universe - This book offers a glimpse of the inner world and immortal realm known to achieved individuals and makes it understandable for students aspiring to a more complete life. BTAOI 0-937064-02-5 218P $14.95

Tao, the Subtle Universal Law - Thoughts and behavior evoke responses from the invisible net of universal energy. This book explains how self-discipline leads to harmony with the universal law. BTAOS 0-937064-01-7 PAPERBACK 208P $12.95

MUSIC AND MISCELLANEOUS

Colored Dust - Sung by Gaille. Poetry by Hua-Ching Ni. - The poetry of Hua-Ching Ni set to music creates a magical sense of transcendence through sound. 37 MINUTES ADUST CASSETTE $10.98, ADUST2 COMPACT DISC $15.95

Poster of Master Lu - Shown on cover of Workbook for Spiritual Development to be used in one's shrine. Image is of Hua-Ching Ni. PMLTP 16" x 22" $10.95

POCKET BOOKLETS

Guide to Your Total Well-Being - Simple useful practices for self-development, aid for your spiritual growth and guidance for all aspects of life. Exercise, food, sex, emotional balancing, meditation. BWELL 0-937064-78-5 PAPERBACK 48P $4.00

Progress Along the Way: Life, Service and Realization - The guiding power of human life is the association between the developed mind and the achieved soul which contains love, rationality, conscience and everlasting value. BPROG 0-937-064-79-3 PAPERBACK 64P $4.00

The Light of All Stars Illuminates the Way - Through generations of searching, various achieved ones found the best application of the Way in their lives. This booklet contains their discovery. BSTAR 0-937064-80-7 48P $4.00

Less Stress More Happiness - Helpful information for identifying and relieving stress in your life including useful techniques such as invocations, breathing and relaxation, meditation, exercise, nutrition and lifestyle balancing. BLESS 0-937064-55-06 48P $3.00

Integral Nutrition - Nutrition is an integral part of a healthy, natural life. Includes information on how to assess your basic body type, food preparation, energetic properties of food, nutrition and digestion. BNUTR 0-937064-84-X 32P $3.00

The Heavenly Way - Straighten Your Way (*Tai Shan Kan Yin Pien*) and The Silent Way of Blessing (*Yin Chia Wen*) are the main sources of inspiration for this booklet that sets the cornerstone for a mature, healthy life. BHEAV 0-937064-03-3 PAPERBACK 42P $2.50

HEALTH AND HEALING

Power of Natural Healing - This book is for anyone wanting to heal themselves or others. Methods include revitalization with acupuncture and herbs, *Tai Chi, Chi Kung (Chi Gong)*, sound, color, movement, visualization and meditation. BHEAL 0-937064-31-9 PAPERBACK 230P $14.95

Attune Your Body with *Dao-In* - The ancient Taoist predecessor to *Tai Chi Chuan*. Performed sitting and lying down, these moves unblock stagnant energy. Includes meditations and massage for a complete integral fitness program. To be used in conjunction with the video. BDAOI 0-937065-40-8 PAPERBACK WITH PHOTO-GRAPHS 144P $14.95

101 Vegetarian Delights - by Lily Chuang and Cathy McNease - A lovely cookbook with recipes as tasty as they are healthy. Features multi-cultural recipes, appendices on Chinese herbs and edible flowers and a glossary of special foods. Over 40 illustrations. B101V 0-937064-13-0 PAPERBACK 176P $12.95

The Tao of Nutrition - by Maoshing Ni, Ph.D., with Cathy McNease, B.S., M.H. - Learn how to take control of your health with good eating. Over 100 common foods are discussed with their energetic properties and therapeutic functions listed. Food therapies for numerous common ailments are also presented. BNUTR 0-937064-66-1 PAPERBACK 214P $14.50

Chinese Vegetarian Delights - by Lily Chuang - An extraordinary collection of recipes based on principles of traditional Chinese nutrition. Meat, sugar, dairy products and fried foods are excluded. BCHIV 0-937064-13-0 PAPERBACK 104P $7.50

Chinese Herbology Made Easy - by Maoshing Ni, Ph.D. - This text provides an overview of Oriental medical theory, in-depth descriptions of each herb category, over 300 black and white photographs, extensive tables of individual herbs for easy reference and an index of pharmaceutical names. BCHIH 0-937064-12-2 PAPERBACK 202P $14.50

Crane Style Chi Gong Book - By Daoshing Ni, Ph.D. - Standing meditative exercises practiced for healing. Combines breathing techniques, movement, and mental imagery to guide the smooth flow of energy. To be used with or without the videotape. BCRAN 0-937064-10-6 SPIRAL-BOUND 55P $10.95

VIDEOTAPES

Natural Living and the Universal Way (VHS) - *New!* - Interview of Hua-Ching Ni in the show "Asian-American Focus" hosted by Lily Chu. Dialogue on common issues of everyday life and practical wisdom. VINTE VHS VIDEO 30 MINUTES $15.95

Movement Arts for Emotional Health (VHS) - *New!* - Interview of Hua-Ching Ni in the show "Asian-American Focus" hosted by Lily Chu. Dialogue on emotional health and energy exercise that are fundamental to health and well-being. VMOVE VHS VIDEO 30 MINUTES $15.95

Attune Your Body with *Dao-In* (VHS) - by Master Hua-Ching Ni. - The ancient Taoist predecessor to *Tai Chi Chuan*. Performed sitting and lying down, these moves unblock stagnant energy. Includes meditations and massage for a complete integral fitness program. VDAOI VHS VIDEO 60 MINUTES $39.95

***T'ai Chi Ch'uan*: An Appreciation (VHS)** - by Hua-Ching Ni. - "Gentle Path," "Sky Journey" and "Infinite Expansion" are three Taoist esoteric styles handed down by highly achieved masters and are shown in an uninterrupted format. Not an instructional video. VAPPR VHS VIDEO 30 MINUTES $24.95

Self-Healing *Chi Gong* (VHS Video) - Strengthen your own self-healing powers. These effective mind-body exercises strengthen and balance each of your five major organ systems. Two hours of practical demonstrations and information lectures. VSHCG VHS VIDEO 120 MINUTES $39.95

Crane Style *Chi Gong* (VHS) - by Dr. Daoshing Ni, Ph.D. - These ancient exercises are practiced for healing purposes. They integrate movement, mental imagery and breathing techniques. To be used with the book. VCRAN VHS VIDEO 120 MINUTES $39.95

Taoist Eight Treasures (VHS) - By Maoshing Ni, Ph.D. - Unique to the Ni family, these 32 exercises open blocks in the energy flow and strengthen one's vitality. Combines stretching, toning and energy conducting with deep breathing Book also available. VEIGH VHS VIDEO 105 MINUTES $39.95

Tai Chi Ch'uan **I & II (VHS)** - By Maoshing Ni, Ph.D. - This Taoist style, called the style of Harmony, is a distillation of the Yang, Chen and Wu styles. It integrates physical movement with internal energy and helps promote longevity and self cultivation. VTAI1 VHS VIDEO PART 1 60 MINUTES $39.95 • VTAI2 VHS VIDEO PART 2 60 MINUTES

AUDIO CASSETTES

Invocations for Health, Longevity and Healing a Broken Heart - By Maoshing Ni, Ph.D. - "Thinking is louder than thunder." This cassette guides you through a series of invocations to channel and conduct your own healing energy and vital force. AINVO AUDIO 30 MINUTES $9.95

Stress Release with Chi Gong - By Maoshing Ni, Ph.D. - This audio cassette guides you through simple breathing techniques that enable you to release stress and tension that are a common cause of illness today. ACHIS AUDIO 30 MINUTES $9.95

Pain Management with Chi Gong - By Maoshing Ni, Ph.D. - Using visualization and deep-breathing techniques, this cassette offers methods for overcoming pain by invigorating your energy flow and unblocking obstructions that cause pain. ACHIP AUDIO 30 MINUTES $9.95

Tao Teh Ching Cassette Tapes - This classic work of Lao Tzu has been recorded in this two-cassette set that is a companion to the book translated by Hua-Ching Ni. Professionally recorded and read by Robert Rudelson. ATAOT 120 MINUTES $12.95

BOOKS IN SPANISH
Tao Teh Ching - En Español. BSPAN 0-937064-92-0 PAPERBACK 112 P $8.95

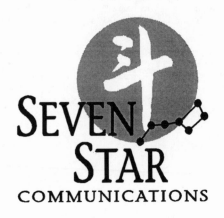

Order Form

Credit Card Information (VISA or MasterCard Only)

Credit Card No. _____

Exp. Date _____

Signature _____

name _____

street address _____

city _____ state _____ zip _____

phone (day) _____ (evening) _____

best time to call _____

Quantity	Price	Title	5 Letter Code	Total

Sub total _____

Sales tax (CA residents only, 8.25%) _____

Shipping (see left) _____

Total Amount Enclosed _____

Shipping Charges

Number of items	Domestic		International			
	UPS Ground	4th Class Book Rate US Mail	Surface US Mail	Air 2 Printed Matter US Mail	Air Parcel Rate US Mail	UPS Int'l Air
First item 1	4.⁵⁰	2.⁰⁰	2.⁵⁰	7.⁵⁰	12.⁰⁰	46.⁰⁰
Each Additional item	0.⁵⁰	0.⁵⁰	1.⁰⁰	5.⁰⁰³	6.⁰⁰	6.⁰⁰

NOTES
1 BOOK OF CHANGES (I CHING) because of weight, counts as 3 items, all other books count as one item each.
2 US Mail Air Printed Matter Table to be used for European destination only. All others use Parcel rate.
3 Limit of 4 items only for this service.

Mail this form with payment
(US funds only) to:
SevenStar Communications
1314 Second Street
Santa Monica, CA 90401 USA

Credit Card Orders:
call **1-800-578-9526**
or fax **310-917-2267**

E-Mail Orders:
taostar@ix.netcom.com
(or call to verify address)

Others Please Call
1-310-576-1901

DELIVERY TIMES
UPS Ground: 7-10 days, Insured
4th Class Book Rate USmail: 5-8 week, Uninsured
Surface US mail (Overseas): 6-9 weeks, Uninsured
Air Printed Matter USmail (Overseas): 2-4 weeks, Uninsured
Air Parcel Rate USmail: 2-4 weeks, Insured
UPS International Air: 4 days, Insured

SEVEN STAR
COMMUNICATIONS

Spiritual Study and Teaching
Through the College of Tao

The College of Tao (COT) and the Union of Tao and Man were formally established in California in the 1970's, yet this tradition is a very broad spiritual culture containing centuries of human spiritual growth. Its central goal is to offer healthy spiritual education to all people. The goal of the school is to help individuals develop themselves for a spiritually developed world. This time-tested school values the spiritual development of each individual self and passes down its guidance and experience.

COT is a school which has no walls. Human society is its classroom. Your own life and service are the class you attend; thus students learn from their lives and from studying the guidance of the Universal Way.

Any interested individual is welcome to join and learn for oneself. The Self-Study Program that is based on Master Ni's books and videotapes gives people who wish to study on their own, or are too far from a teacher, an opportunity to study the Universal Way. The outline for the Self-Study Program is given in the book *The Golden Message*. If you choose, a Correspondence Course is also available.

A Mentor is any individual who is spiritually self-responsible and who is a model of a healthy and complete life. A Mentor may serve as a teacher for general society and people with a preliminary interest in spiritual development. To be certified to teach, a Mentor must first register with the USIW and follow the Mentor Service Handbook, which was written by Mentors. It is recommended that all prospective Mentors use the Correspondence Course or self-study program to educate themselves, but they may also learn directly from other Mentors. COT offers special seminars taught only to Mentors.

If you are interested in the Integral Way of Life Correspondence Course, please write: College of Tao, PO Box 1222, El Prado, NM 87529 USA.

- -

If you would like more information about the USIW and classes in your area, please send the following form to: USIW, PO Box 28993, Atlanta, GA 30358-0993

❐   I wish to be put on the mailing list of the USIW to be notified of educational activities.

❐   I wish to receive a list of Registered Mentors teaching in my area or country.

❐   I am interested in joining /forming a study group in my area.

❐   I am interested in becoming a Mentor of the USIW.

Name:_____

Address:_____

City:_____State:_____Zip:_____

Country:_____

Herbs Used by Ancient Masters

The pursuit of everlasting youth or immortality throughout human history is an innate human desire. Long ago, Chinese esoteric Taoists went to the high mountains to contemplate nature, strengthen their bodies, empower their minds and develop their spirit. From their studies and cultivation, they gave China alchemy and chemistry, herbology and acupuncture, the I Ching, astrology, martial arts and T'ai Chi Ch'uan, Chi Gong and many other useful kinds of knowledge.

Most important, they handed down in secrecy methods for attaining longevity and spiritual immortality. There were different levels of approach; one was to use a collection of food herb formulas that were only available to highly achieved Taoist masters. They used these food herbs to increase energy and heighten vitality. This treasured collection of herbal formulas remained within the Ni family for centuries.

Now, through Traditions of Tao, the Ni family makes these foods available for you to use to assist the foundation of your own positive development. It is only with a strong foundation that expected results are produced from diligent cultivation.

As a further benefit, in concert with the Taoist principle of self-sufficiency, Traditions of Tao offers the food herbs along with SevenStar Communication's publications in a distribution opportunity for anyone serious about financial independence.

Send to: *Traditions of Tao*
              1314 Second Street #200
              Santa Monica, CA 90401

Please send me a Traditions of Tao brochure.

Name _____

Address _____

City _____ *State* _____ *Zip* _____

Phone (day) _____ *(evening)* _____

Yo San University of Traditional Chinese Medicine

"Not just a medical career, but a life-time commitment to raising one's spiritual standard."

Thank you for your support and interest in our publications and services. It is by your patronage that we continue to offer you the practical knowledge and wisdom from this venerable Taoist tradition.

Because of your sustained interest in natural health, in January 1989 we formed Yo San University of Traditional Chinese Medicine, a non-profit educational institution under the direction of founder Master Ni, Hua-Ching. Yo San University is the continuation of 38 generations of Ni family practitioners who handed down knowledge and wisdom from father to son. Its purpose is to train and graduate practitioners of the highest caliber in Traditional Chinese Medicine, which includes acupuncture, herbology and spiritual development.

We view Traditional Chinese Medicine as the application of spiritual development. Its foundation is the spiritual capability to know life, diagnose a person's problem and cure it. We teach students how to care for themselves and others, emphasizing the integration of traditional knowledge and modern science. Yo San University offers a complete accredited Master's degree program approved by the California State Department of Education that provides an excellent education in Traditional Chinese Medicine and meets all requirements for state licensure. Federal financial aid and scholarships are available.

We invite you to inquire into our university for a creative and rewarding career as a holistic physician. Classes are also open to persons interested only in self-enrichment. For more information, please fill out the form below and send it to:

> Yo San University of Traditional Chinese Medicine
> 1314 Second Street
> Santa Monica, CA 90401 U.S.A.

❏　Please send me information on the Masters degree program in Traditional Chinese Medicine.

❏　Please send me information on health workshops and seminars.

❏　Please send me information on continuing education for acupuncturists and health professionals.

Name _____

*Address*_____

*City*_____*State*_____*Zip*_____

*Phone (day)*_____*(evening)*_____

Master Ni's work is an enormous treasure I am using to restore myself. His teachings support my *T'ai Chi* practice, which I began 5 years ago to improve my condition due to spinal column damage. My health improved greatly and a new life began.

Urs Bitzi, Mund, Germany

Along with acupuncture and herbs, the Eight Treasures video has improved my body, mind and spirit 100%. Miracles do happen. Now I move forward to *Dao-In*. Give my respects to Master Ni and his sons for sharing a part of their knowledge with me.

Sharron Lee Reynolds, Montreal, Canada

Recently I purchased your video of *Dao-In*. It is very useful and I appreciate its simplicity. I am looking forward to receiving the book that goes along with it. I have a ligament injury on my right leg/knee area so can't do standing exercises for long periods of time or even take long walks now, so the tape is especially helpful to keep the muscles exercised and as general fitness.

Also, as a meditation and *Chi Gong* practitioner and student of Taoist material, I really appreciate having my experience verified by what is written in Master Ni's books.

Robert Walther, Aptos, California

Index